IN TOUCH

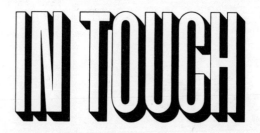

IN TOUCH

Aids and Services
for Blind and Partially Sighted People

Margaret Ford and Thena Heshel

Illustrations by Patricia Capon

British Broadcasting Corporation

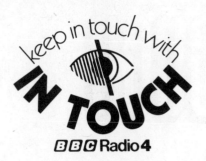

In Touch is a programme of news, comment and information for visually handicapped people which is broadcast weekly on Radio 4. In addition to the programme, the *In Touch* team produces a free quarterly bulletin summarising the information broadcast; this is also available in braille from the Scottish Braille Press which prints the braille edition of this book. There is also an off-air phone-in to give blind listeners a chance to pass on comments, suggestions or queries to the *In Touch* team. Details of broadcast and phone-in times are given in *Radio Times*. Since its beginning in 1961, the programme has been made and presented by blind broadcasters and journalists.

The first presenter of In Touch *was David Scott Blackhall, who worked on the programme from its inception until shortly before his death in September 1981. This edition is dedicated to his memory. We hope that the book will continue to aid all those who battle daily as he did to overcome the many problems which beset people with little or no sight.*

Published by the
British Broadcasting Corporation, 35 Marylebone High Street, London W1M 4AA
ISBN 0 563 17907 4
First published 1973, Revised edition 1977, Third edition 1982
© British Broadcasting Corporation 1982
Printed in England by Whitstable Litho Ltd, Millstrood Road, Whitstable, Kent

Contents

Foreword

When we produced the first 'In Touch' handbook in 1973, it was an attempt to put together in permanent form all the information on aids, services and equipment which had been broadcast on the *In Touch* programme, which is BBC Radio 4's regular weekly programme for visually handicapped people. Our intention was to provide not only blind and partially sighted people, but also those setting out to help them, with a guide to what is available and where to find it. This third edition has information about a much wider range of aids and equipment; but while this is an indication that more is available to help the blind, it is unfortunately not true that blind people are now receiving a better service. The preface to the first edition stated that one thing blind people had in common, apart from their lack of sight, was lack of information about the help available to them. Nine years later we are able to describe in this book developments costing hundreds of thousands of pounds, which have resulted in equipment that will convert print into sound – but the *In Touch* team still regularly gets queries from blind listeners who are unable to find out locally how to join the Talking Book Library or where to get a white stick!

There are two factors which contribute to this situation. The specialist social worker for the blind is an increasingly rare bird: the latest surveys show that the ratio of local authority specialists to registered blind people ranges from 1:100 to 1:1000, and the abolition of the full-time specialist post for the visually handicapped within the social work department of the DHSS bodes ill for any future improvement of this situation. But in addition to the dearth of specialists, there is another factor. The majority of blind people are old: we live in an ageing society and visual handicap comes primarily in extreme old age. Many of these old people do not get registered, and are therefore not likely to be in touch with the relevant services. If their needs are going to be met, those concerned with the care of the elderly will need to become more aware of the needs of the visually handicapped. As our contribution to this growing need, we have added a new chapter on the care of the elderly, which may be as relevant to those who work for organisations – such as Age Concern, the WRVS or the Red Cross – which are in regular contact with the elderly as it is to those whose prime concern is for the blind.

As always, when we have surveyed the services for the visually handicapped, we have been heartened by the generosity and kindly intentions of so many people and agencies. But it is apparent that many needs are still unmet. The blind are debarred from statutory financial benefits such as the mobility and attendance allowances unless they have the misfortune to suffer also from further handicaps. The 1981 budget did double the blind person's income tax allowance, but only a very small number of blind people are in the happy position of having an income large enough to pay tax on it. Government shows little sign yet of following the example of other countries in making statutory provision for a blindness allowance, and recent cuts in social services' budgets mean that services on which many blind people rely are being reduced.

The cuts in public spending have been justified by government on the grounds that reserves of voluntary help are available. The blind are in the fortunate position of possessing affluent and powerful voluntary organisations, and these have indeed pioneered many valuable services. But needs change faster than institutions and charities which have the greatest appeal to the public do not necessarily meet the greatest need. The Guide Dogs for the Blind Association, whose assets totalled around £20 million in 1981, do sterling work for Britain's 3,000 guide dog owners, but, unlike their Australian counterparts, offer no alternative mobility training with long canes or sonic aids which could benefit many more thousands of blind people and supplement the inadequacies of local authority services.

St Dunstan's, founded in 1919 to provide for the war-blinded, is the wealthiest of the blind charities but in 1981 there were only 998 war-blinded men and women living in Britain. In 1981, St Dunstan's income from legacies and investments was nearly £4 million and its assets were valued at nearly £28 million. Under the chairmanship of its founder, Lord Fraser, St Dunstan's in 1948 resolved to make grants to any charity for the Blind 'whose objects, or any of whose objects is to render services which are or may be of benefit to war-blinded persons' and subsequently St Dunstan's contributed to the Talking Book Service and the National Mobility Centre as well as some research projects. But now St Dunstan's seems surprisingly reluctant to contribute to projects which help the blind in general. In 1981, only £8,876 was given to other charities for the blind and a mere £1,757 contributed for research – yet £1.3 million was put into St Dunstan's reserves – a figure that would go a long way towards financing the recording and distribution of a national daily – or weekly – newspaper, which would bring great pleasure to many blind people, including St Dunstaners.

It is not generally appreciated that none of the journals or magazines sold by the millions at every bookstall are nationally available on tape for the blind. The Talking Book Library attempts to provide a service for 54,000 blind people, but has less than 4,000 titles in its catalogue. The latest advance in recording techniques, announced late in 1981 by the Foundation for Audio Research, means that it would now be possible to record full length novels on to only two C90 cassettes for playback on a new-style recording machine which could also play ordinary cassettes. This could be the key that would open to the blind population a wealth of literature never before thought accessible. But it would need several millions of pounds to get underway; and millions of pounds lie idle in the reserves of blind charities.

But fortunately it is not always essential to pass laws or raise thousands of pounds to effect some improvement in a blind person's life. Our new chapter on ways of helping is designed to show some of the ways in which ordinary people without specialist skills can help. An ability to listen with empathy, to convey information clearly and to know when to offer help tactfully and appropriately are the gifts needed. Fortunately, these talents are not confined to experts – we hope that this book will be of use to those people in the helping agencies and in the community, who would like to 'help the Blind' but are deterred because they have no specialist knowledge. We hope, with the help of the information given here, people will be heartened by the amount of kindliness there is available once the appropriate door has been knocked upon, and the person or agency that meets a blind person's particular need has been finally tracked down.

The *In Touch* team will do its best to help by providing information about aids, services and equipment on the programme and for those who want to have a permanent record, there are quarterly bulletins which summarise the broadcast information. In addition, the *In Touch* team can be contacted on the weekly off-air phone-in to deal with comments or queries arising from the programme.

We would like to thank the *In Touch* team of blind reporters and presenters, Peter White, Jane Finnis, Kevin Mulhern and Hannah Wright, who provide an on-going critical consumer view of what is provided for the visually handicapped. It is their work, supported by the patient and painstaking research of our assistant Anne Theak-stone, which has laid the foundation for this book. In addition, we are particularly grateful for the advice of Nick Beard, Elizabeth Chapman, Stephen Clive, David Ellis, Valerie Scarr, Joan Shields and Dr Michael Wolffe, and would like to thank Keeler Optical Products for permitting us to reproduce their Word Chart.

Finally, our thanks to the many blind listeners whose letters, comments and criticisms are a constant stimulation to us all. Often it is blind people themselves who come up with easy solutions to everyday problems and some of these hints are reproduced in this book. No doubt other ideas and suggestions will continue to flow, and we will do our best to reflect them through "In Touch".

Thena Heshel
Margaret Ford

The end – or the beginning?

The words 'registered as blind' reverberate in the mind as the final sentence – the end of the story. Shock, disbelief, grief, resentment and plain fear mingle together as gradually the realisation dawns on the listener that this label is personal. For some the words may come initially almost as a relief – they represent the end of years of apprehension, of hopes raised and dashed again, of life measured out in terms of visits to the eye clinic. But when hopes are extinguished, even those years of anxiety can be yearned for as being more desirable than reality. For the very elderly, where loss of vision has gradually accompanied the slow fading of other faculties and is accepted as part of an inevitable ageing process, the blow is softened. But even the very aged can grieve for lost faculties, and for them the fear that this loss will also inevitably deprive them of their independence may be realised.

There is no magic formula which enables anyone to come to terms with visual loss. The only easy thing about the phrase 'accepting your blindness' is the way it trips off the tongue of would-be helpers; all have to work out for themselves their own unique way through this 'dark night of the soul'. And to that task they will bring the experience of their whole sighted life and their whole personality. Their strengths and weaknesses, skills and failings, their capacity for making relationships, feelings about themselves and their ideas of what blindness is and how blind people behave, all influence their adjustment. For some, the journey is long and difficult; for others, to the outsider at least, the way seems to be smoother. The key seems to lie not in the severity of the handicap, but in the personal resources and the lifestyle of the individual. An inability to read may be the most grievous deprivation imaginable to one person, but dismissed as a minor handicap by another. Nor is there such a thing as a 'good adjustment'; that can only be assessed with regard to each individual. The husband who was always waited on by his wife before losing his sight can hardly be classed as being overdependent when he insists she now ties his laces as well as fetching his shoes.

Loss of sight has sometimes been likened to bereavement. Certainly, a newly blinded person needs plenty of opportunity to talk about his or her deprivation. It is no kindness to try to ignore the predicament and to laboriously avoid mentioning topics that refer too directly to the handicap. 'How much can you see?' is not necessarily a tactless question; it gives an opportunity for a verbal assessment of the situation. Encouragement to talk about the failed operation, or the treatment at the clinic, is helpful. Just putting into words that confused impression of anxious and perhaps painful weeks in strange surroundings helps to impose an order and pattern on those events, and this is in itself reassuring. It may well be that blame for the failure of the treatment is attached to some entirely innocent person, or loss of sight may be attributed to some innocuous incident or set of circumstances many years ago; to identify a scapegoat is one way of dealing with resentment and aggression. In times of stress, it is no kindness to shatter such illusions. Given time, most people can divert these feelings into more productive channels. The force that makes a person curse fate is an invaluable ally when it also gives the determination to take that first unnerving walk out of doors with only a white stick for company.

But there is more to adjusting to blindness than coping with the actual vision loss. In many ways that battle is the easiest to fight, once energy, will and initiative have been harnessed to the task. The hardest part of visual handicap is the barrier it places between the blind person and the world at large.

Because blindness is such a distinctive handicap, people tend to see the handicap rather than the person; and immediately conversation is inhibited, whilst they unnecessarily grope for synonyms for 'look' and 'see'. The relationship is made more difficult because the handicap of blindness has its own special mystique that has grown up around it from the earliest times, and we tend to treat a blind person as someone quite different from ourselves. It is extremely hard to remember that the blind person is exactly the same person as before sight was lost. Acute hearing, extra sensitive touch or even extraordinary virtue is not suddenly acquired. That someone has lit a cigarette does not mean that a feat equivalent to walking on water has been performed.

Most people, if asked what qualities were characteristic of the blind, would put bravery, courage and cheerfulness on their list and probably helplessness and dependency would be there too. It is easy to forget that, while still sighted, the blind person probably had much the same ideas. An already damaged self-image is, therefore, undergoing another battering as the realisation dawns of *not* feeling any of those virtues – of being just anxious, frightened or plain miserable, with apparently a built-in ability to create a disaster area with every unguarded movement. Helplessness and dependency are very real emotions, but they may be accompanied by an uneasy feeling that blind people are well known to be extremely grateful for all the help given them – why, then, is this resentment also felt?

It has been argued that blindness is, above everything else, a learned social role. In other words, blind people behave in the way expected of them. If everybody expects them to be helpless and dependent, then this they will be. Friends and relatives naturally want to help and their almost instinctive reaction will be 'let me do that for you'. But it is essential to offer help and encouragement according to the blind individual's own very unique needs, not according to the needs of the imaginary typical blind person. If someone has always been very independent, it is essential that efforts are directed to finding ways to encourage this. It may be agony to watch fumbling; 'helping' in this sense is emotionally far more demanding on the 'helper' than actually doing the job for the blind person would be. Kindness can be cruel when it tries to relieve the blind person of all anxiety and responsibility. Nor should losing one sense lead inevitably to loss of status. The fact that people have lost their sight does not mean that all decisions should be made for them. It merely means that they must be given information verbally, which previously they would have gathered with their eyes, so that they can have the data on which to make decisions.

That is why this is primarily an information handbook. It does not pretend to be able to solve every visually handicapped person's problems, but only to show some of the ways by which very ordinary visually handicapped people have found that they have again been able to lead useful, interesting and satisfying lives. It is hoped that newly visually handicapped readers will be able to learn from this experience, and to adapt it to their own needs as they come to terms with their handicap in their own way. But it is also hoped that sighted readers will receive the message that the real need of the blind is not a sheltered seat in a scented garden but the opportunity to take their place in the hurly-burly of everyday life.

2 How to get help

How much can you see?

What is blindness?
The lay conception of blindness as total loss of sight differs radically from the definition given by the National Assistance Act of 1948. A person need not be unable to see at all in order to be registered as blind. Nor does registration imply that sight is going to deteriorate until light can no longer be distinguished from dark. In fact, about 85 per cent of people registered as blind have some useful vision. Generally speaking a person is 'blind' if, he or she can read, only at three metres distance, letters on a chart that a person with normal sight can read at sixty metres distance. But someone able to see much more than this may also be registered as blind if the field of vision is severely restricted; a typical example is a person who can see the clock face on the mantelpiece but not the ornaments on either side of it. The definition of blindness for the purpose of registration is 'so blind as to be unable to perform any work for which eyesight is essential'.

What is partial sight?
Broadly speaking, this term covers those whose sight, though poor, is not bad enough for them technically to be registered as blind. Partially sighted people may be able to distinguish objects no better than the 'blind', but the field of vision may not be so limited; or they may be able to see more clearly than a 'blind' person, but only within a restricted field. Partially sighted people are 'substantially and permanently handicapped by congenitally defective vision of a substantial and permanently handicapping character', or have suffered from an illness or injury that has caused 'defective vision of a substantial or permanently handicapping character'. People registered as partially sighted come within the scope of local authority services for the blind or handicapped, but this does not entitle them to as many financial benefits as those registered blind (see Chapter 3, *Money*).

What is visual handicap?
This phrase is now generally used instead of 'blindness' or 'partial sight' because it gives a clearer indication of the person's difficulties. The term 'severe visual handicap' is usually reserved for those who

retain only very little useful vision. In this book 'visual handicap' will always be preferred to 'blindness' or 'partial sight', except in those instances when the service mentioned is exclusive to one or other category of registration.

Registration

A register of the blind and partially-sighted people living within its area is kept by every county council, metropolitan district council and each London borough. Registration is voluntary on the part of the visually handicapped, but the local authority will only register them if a consultant ophthalmologist, who is a doctor (*not* an optician) has completed a form (known as the BD8) reporting on a patient's sight, and has recommended registration in either category of visual handicap. If the specialist recommends registration as partially sighted, but considers that it is likely that the patient's sight will deteriorate, and that there would be 'benefit from training for employment or other services appropriate to blind people' this will be indicated on the BD8.

The same procedure is followed for the registration of children. Proposals to replace the BD8 for children under sixteen years by a 'notification of significant visual handicap' which would take into account both near and distance vision are under active consideration but, in 1981, not yet implemented.

Why register?

In order to qualify for the services provided by both central and local government, and to enlist the help of the voluntary societies.

How to get on the register

Anyone being treated at hospital for a serious eye condition will probably find that the specialist will discuss registration if his or her sight is sufficiently poor, and will also notify the social services department of the relevant local authority. A social worker will then visit to discuss the services available and, if this is wanted, will ask the specialist to complete a BD8. Once this has been accepted by the local authority, the patient's name is added to the appropriate register. There may be a time lag, but the effective date of registration is that on the BD8, an important point to remember when a newly registered blind person is claiming income tax relief or supplementary benefit.

19

If patients feel they have neither the opportunity nor the courage to discuss registration with their eye specialist, the hospital medical social worker will be very willing to talk the matter over with them informally and, if necessary, start the registration procedure for them.

People not attending hospital should contact their local social services department. Area offices can be found in most towns and the local town hall, Citizen's Advice Bureau or library should be able to give the address. If appropriate, a social worker will arrange a registration examination by a consultant ophthalmologist. Examination at home can be arranged for the housebound, and transport to hospital can be provided for those unable to use public transport. The examination costs the patient nothing; the Area Health Authority pays the specialist's fees. If the patient should disagree with the specialist's recommendation – for example, feeling that the blind register rather than that for the partially sighted would be more appropriate, the local authority can be asked to refer the case for an independent examination to the Ophthalmic Referee Service provided in their respective areas by the Southern and Western Regional Association, the North Regional Association, the Scottish National Federation and the Wales Council.

Who will help?

Central government services
Central government is responsible for deciding the main financial benefits (Chapter 3, *Money*) and, through the Manpower Services Commission, resettlement and retraining services for visually handicapped people seeking employment. Registered blind people are entitled to vote by post at all local and parliamentary elections. Application forms for postal votes can be obtained from the Electoral Registration Officer. Alternatively, a blind voter may ask the help of the Presiding Officer at the polling station, or take a close relative, or a companion who has a vote in the same constituency, to help. No companion may act for more than two blind people at any one election.

Local government services
Section 29 of the National Assistance Act, 1948, as amended by virtue of the Local Government Act 1972, empowers a local authority to

make the following arrangements for the welfare of substantially and permanently handicapped people, including the blind and partially sighted.

*1   to provide a social work service and such advice and support as may be needed for people living in their own homes or elsewhere;

*2   to provide, whether at centres or elsewhere, facilities for social rehabilitation and adjustment to disability including assistance in overcoming limitations of mobility or communication;

*3   to provide, whether at centres or elsewhere, facilities for occupational, social, cultural and recreational activities and, where appropriate, the making of payments to persons for work undertaken by them;

4   to provide hostels for persons undertaking training or employment and to provide holiday homes;

5   to provide free or subsidised travel for all or any persons registered with the council as handicapped;

6   to assist in finding suitable supportive lodgings;

7   to contribute to the cost of employing a warden on welfare functions in warden-assisted housing schemes;

8   to provide warden services for occupiers of private housing;

9   to arrange, where appropriate, for the provision of any of the above services by another local authority, or voluntary organisation;

*10   to arrange for the keeping of registers of persons to whom section 29 applies.

Although this means that local authorities have the power to do all these things, they are only *required* to make arrangements for the services listed under points 1, 2, 3 and 10. In other words, the starred services are mandatory; the others are permissive.

In addition, under the Chronically Sick and Disabled Persons Act, 1970, *if it considers it necessary*, the local authority must help substantially and permanently handicapped people (a phrase which again includes the blind and partially sighted) with the following services:

1   practical help and adaptations in their homes;

2   radio, television or similar recreational facilities at home;

3   outside recreational and education facilities, and help in making use of them such as providing means of travel;

4   holidays;

5   meals at home or elsewhere;

6   a telephone and any special equipment needed to use it.

The local authority therefore has a duty to advise and help visually handicapped people with, for example, improved lighting in the home

– but only if it is satisfied that there is real need for such help. The local authority may charge for these services, though often simple aids are loaned free.

The provision of telephones especially has caused much disappointment, as most visually handicapped people consider they 'need' one. As a result, local authorities tend to follow nationally agreed guidelines to decide whether a telephone is a necessity. The person must live alone, or be frequently left alone, or be housebound, and also require a telephone for medical and social reasons. Only when all these conditions are met, and the client has also been assessed as needing financial help, will most local authorities consider a telephone to be necessary, and therefore something that they have a duty to provide. Some local authorities, however, interpret 'need' more generously than others. For example, in 1978/79 the amount spent by local authorities on telephone rental and installation in England and Wales ranged from £16 per 1,000 population to £616. The total number of installations rose slightly in that period, though some local authorities cut back on the number of rentals paid.

Social services departments
Most of the local government services mentioned above are supplied through local authority social services departments, though some have delegated their powers (or certain aspects of them) to voluntary societies who act as their agents. In all cases, however, the local social worker at the local social services area office is the key person to contact.

Depending on the staffing situation, a visually handicapped person may find quite a range of social workers. The first visit may be made by a generic social worker, that is, a social worker trained to help with a wide range of problems but who has not specialised in one particular handicap such as blindness.

He or she may be referred to a mobility officer, who has been trained to teach blind people to move about safely and confidently, both indoors and out. Or a technical officer may come and visit, to teach communication and daily living skills (reading, writing, cooking, cleaning and simple sewing). Sometimes technical and mobility skills are combined in one person, who may then be called a rehabilitation officer.

Many visually handicapped people would say, however, that their problem was not that they saw three workers, but that they never seemed to be visited by even one! It is probably unrealistic to expect regular social visits, but visually handicapped people should not hesitate to make their needs known at their local area office. Constructive suggestions as to how a local service could be improved are always welcome. Indeed, one local authority at least has its own 'consumer group' of visually handicapped people to advise and comment on needs and services as they themselves experience them.

Complaints procedure: People who feel that their local authority has handled their request for help incompetently, unjustifiably slowly, or that it has failed to take relevant considerations into account, should complain, in the first instance, to the department or authority involved. Then, if the matter cannot be resolved, they should approach their local councillor. In the last resort, they may lodge these types of complaints, through their councillor, with the local Ombudsman. It should be remembered, however, that the Ombudsman deals only with complaints that injustice has been caused by a fault in the way the local authority has done something, or if it has not done something it should have done. He has no power to question the action of a local authority just because the complainant does not agree with it.

National voluntary organisations

The Royal National Institute for the Blind, one third of whose council members are themselves blind, aims to be 'the helping hand to all Britain's blind'. It provides education facilities, rehabilitation centres, employment services, homes, hostels, holiday hotels, braille and Moon literature, talking books, training for mobility instructors, supports research projects and designs, and produces special apparatus and equipment. The latter is sold at concession prices to all registered blind and partially sighted people in this country, to local voluntary societies for the blind, and to sighted individuals buying on behalf of the blind. An illustrated catalogue (or its braille equivalent) is free on request, together with price lists which are updated twice a year. In conjunction with the American Foundation for the Blind an *International Directory of Aids and Appliances for Blind and Visually Impaired Persons* is compiled and revised periodically and can be obtained in braille and inkprint. The RNIB will obtain, on request from customers, items listed which are not normally available in this country. Anyone wishing to make comments or suggestions regarding RNIB goods should write in the first instance to the Director General who will forward letters, where appropriate, to a consumers' committee which consists of twenty blind people, half of whom are nominated by organisations for the blind. The Institute's journal *The New Beacon* is issued monthly in braille and inkprint.

The Partially Sighted Society was founded in 1973, mainly as a result of pressure from the parents of partially sighted children. It is concerned with the welfare of people of all ages with poor sight, and has branches in twenty areas of the country. *Oculus*, a bi-monthly magazine in large print, is available free to members, and to others on payment. Advice and guidance can be given on all aspects of partial sight and the Society has committees looking at the problems of employment, education, mobility, social services and technical aids. Details of membership and an application form are available on request.

Other major national organisations include *St Dunstan's* who are responsible for the life-long care of men and women blinded whilst serving in HM Forces and the *National Library for the Blind* which provides a postal library service in braille and Moon. *The Catholic Blind Institute* and the *Jewish Blind Society* provide special services for those of their faiths, but are always ready to share their expertise with others. *The Guide Dogs for the Blind Association* provides training and guide dogs for all blind people in the United Kingdom able to benefit from their services. *The National Deaf-Blind Helpers' League* provides special service, help, support and encouragement for the deaf-blind adults while the *National Association for the Deaf-Blind and Rubella Handicapped* exists to serve the needs of children, young people and their parents.

Local voluntary societies
A few local authorities continue to ask voluntary societies to act as their agents for all their responsibilities under section 29 of the National Assistance Act. Other voluntary societies arrange only recreational facilities, the provision of craft material, and the marketing of finished products. But all societies are under considerable pressure to increase their services and also to act as friendly and neighbourly visitors for the blind.

Inevitably, the standard of voluntary service varies from one district to another. In some areas, there may be little more than an occasional social or outing, a Christmas gift or a Christmas party. In others, the voluntary society has its own purpose-built premises, with a daily programme of education and recreation. Some societies supply a dial-a-reader service, others a 'phone-in' service; some employ full-time visitors to visit housebound or lonely blind people regularly. Almost every service one can think of is provided somewhere by a voluntary society.

If a visually handicapped person happens to live in the right place it may be possible to join groups for hiking, yachting, bell-ringing, choral singing, pottery or Old Time Dancing. A Christmas gift may be £1 or there might be £12 in a Christmas card from the voluntary society. One society will give fuel grants in winter, another will provide blankets, while a third will provide a braille clock. It is not unknown for a voluntary society to repair a leaking roof, replace a lost purse, decorate a room, insulate a roof, or supply an electric blanket. By various means to varied extents, they meet the very varied needs of local people. The address of the nearest voluntary society can be obtained from the local social services department, or on request from the RNIB. *The Directory of Agencies for the Blind*, available from the RNIB in braille and inkprint, lists all voluntary societies.

Self-help groups
The majority of the agencies so far mentioned are run mainly by sighted people; blind representatives on their committees are generally very much in the minority. Two major organisations, however, are run for the blind and by the blind.

The National League of the Blind and Disabled of Great Britain and Ireland: This has 60 branches and six District Councils. Any blind or partially sighted person over 16 years of age can join; its membership is extended also to sighted disabled people employed in sheltered workshops. Affiliated to the TUC and the Labour Party, as well as to the International Federation of the Blind, it is the trade union for blind workshop employees, who account for 60 per cent of its membership, but its concern is for the blind population as a whole. At present the League is engaged on a campaign to draw attention to the 10 per cent of blind people who, registered as being available for work, are unemployed. It is concerned at the high cost of specialist equipment, and believes that if research were funded on an EEC basis costs would eventually be reduced as the market for such equipment would then be very much greater. The League has two periodicals: *The Horizon*, a braille bi-monthly and its inkprint equivalent *The Blind Advocate*, a quarterly which is also available on tape through the Tape Recording Society for the Blind.

The National Federation of the Blind: Open to all blind and partially sighted people over the age of 16. It has about thirty branches and a postal branch for those not within easy reach of a local branch. It offers the fellowship of other blind people and a means of voicing the views of blind people on all questions affecting them. It campaigns for a handicap allowance for all blind people, the integrated education of visually handicapped children in ordinary schools, better job opportunities and social services, free transport, the provision of telephones and a safer and more accessible environment. It is anxious to increase participation by blind people in committees providing services for the blind. A quarterly journal *Viewpoint* is published in braille and inkprint, and recorded on tape.

Special interest groups
Where a number of visually handicapped people are employed in a profession, self-help groups generally emerge. However, these groups are also useful sources of advice for newly registered blind people considering entering the professions or trades involved.

   The Society of Blind Lawyers, the *Clerics Group*, the *British Computer Association of the Blind*, the *Association of Blind Chartered Physiotherapists*, the *Association of Blind Piano Tuners* all exist to protect and further the interests of their members and keep them up to date, by brailled or taped information, with developments in their respective fields. The *Association of Visually Handicapped Telephonists* was formed with the aim of helping its members keep abreast of the rapidly changing technical development in switchboard design and to obtain suitable employment, and the *Visually Handicapped Office Workers Group* provides a forum for secretaries and office workers to discuss developments in office technology and career problems. The *Association of Blind and Partially Sighted Teachers and Students* enables its members to exchange ideas and to bring their collective experience as consumers to bear on the development of services to meet their needs. The *Circle of Guide Dog Owners* exists to provide opportunities for exchange of ideas between guide dog owners and to enable the consumer's voice to be heard by the *Guide Dogs for the Blind Association*.

Patient centred groups
With the many causes of visual handicap, it is surprising to find only two associations of sufferers from a particular type of blindness.

The British Retinitis Pigmentosa Society: circulates information quarterly in large print, braille and cassette on medical and social aspects of the disease, and members meet socially both for mutual support and to raise funds for research. An eye donor scheme, set up in 1980, is already advancing research into the causes and treatment of retinitis pigmentosa (RP).

International Glaucoma Association: presses for better facilities for the management of glaucoma and gives advice to patients on the problems they may meet. It aims to prevent loss of sight from glaucoma throughout the world.

Professional associations
The *Association for the Education and Welfare of the Visually Handicapped*, the *National Association of Orientation and Mobility Instructors* and the *National Association of Technical Officers for the Blind* are all relatively small organisations representing the interests of professionals engaged in education and welfare, mobility and technical work respectively. In 1979 a new organisation *The Visual Impairment Association* was formed with the aim of working towards an organisation which would encompass all workers with visually impaired people.
The many local voluntary societies in England and Wales are grouped together and represented on and by the *Southern and Western Regional Association*, the *Wales Council* and the *Northern Regional Association for the Blind*. A bi-annual journal is issued: *The Inter-Regional Review*, available in braille and inkprint.

Access to help
Anybody reading this far will not need convincing that the network of services available for the visually handicapped has the doubtful dis-

tinction of being the most complex of any of the services of the handicapped. Nor does it seem likely that it will become simpler. Services for the blind are rooted in the nineteenth century; and, inevitably, well-established organisations – although still doing sterling work – tend to lack flexibility. New groups, therefore, emerge to meet new needs. It is sad that the people they exist to serve are the very ones who are most likely to be confused by a multiplicity of sources of help. To try to overcome this, in recent years a number of local voluntary societies and social services departments have produced their own guides to services in their areas. The best are written simply and succinctly, in large clear print and manage to convey a warm and welcoming atmosphere as well as basic information. Readers should enquire from their local social services department and/or voluntary agency if such a guide is available for their area. If so, it would be an invaluable companion to this book. A simple free guide to services by the state entitled *Help for Handicapped People* (HB1) is widely available in social security offices, social services departments, Citizens Advice Bureaux and other similar agencies. It can be obtained free, in braille, from the RNIB. A companion booklet *Aids for the Disabled* (HB2) is a useful reference point for professional workers concerned with services for the disabled and their families.

Opportunities to handle the wide range of equipment mentioned in this book have until recently been virtually non-existent, though RNIB equipment can always be examined on a 'sale or return' basis at branch offices in Liverpool, Manchester, Leeds, Cambridge, Hove, Bristol, Cardiff, Stirling and Belfast; and the whole range is stocked at *224 Great Portland Street, London, W1N 6AA.*

Spurred on by the popularity of the annual *See By Touch* exhibitions initiated by the British Retinitis Pigmentosa Society, a growing number of voluntary societies and some local authorities have now established their own permanent displays. The Strathclyde Resource Centre for the Blind in Glasgow is a notable example. The *In Touch* team has visited different parts of the country mounting displays and demonstrations of items described in the programme and, as resources permit, it is hoped to continue this service from time to time.

Further Reading
The Eye in Health and Disease (1978). Northern Regional Association

28

for the Blind. A simple guide to the eye and explanation of terms used in the BD8.

Chronically Sick and Disabled Persons Act, 1970. A guide to help you overcome some hurdles. Disablement Income Group.

Help for People with Failing Sight (1981). Royal National Institute for the Blind. Free pamphlet.

★ *The rain-warning device (made by the RNIB) is used by one lady to contact her neighbour in case of need. She places it by an open window, wets the top so that it emits its shrill alarm and her neighbour knows it is a signal for help.*
(Lilian Jones, Shrewsbury)

★ *A useful way to remember telephone numbers is to substitute letters of the alphabet for the numbers, that is, the letters A to I for 1 to 9 and the letter O for zero. It is then quite easy to construct a phrase using the letters. An example would be 6057 giving the letters FOEG and making the phrase Fine Old English Gentleman.*
(David Scott Blackhall)

★ *When buying stamps ask the counter-clerk to place them the right way up, then fold over the top left-hand corner of the left-hand stamp. Leave this to be used last, and you will always know that you are sticking stamps on letters correctly.*
(Maurice Derby, Bristol)

3 Money

There is no automatic State 'blind pension'. At present, the only allowances that resemble one are the pensions awarded if blindness is due to service in the armed forces and the industrial disablement benefit paid when blindness results from an accident at work. But blindness rarely arises from either of these causes. The Royal National Institute for the Blind, the National League of the Blind and the National Federation of the Blind are all campaigning for a blindness allowance to help meet the extra costs incurred through visual disability.

The only automatic financial help for a registered blind person is a reduction of £1.25 in the cost of the sound and television receiving licence (see page 164), a few travel and parking fee concessions (see page 194), some postal concessions (see page 76) and a free licence for a guide dog.

Visually handicapped people are, of course, eligible for National Insurance benefits in the same way as the rest of the population provided they have fulfilled the necessary contribution requirements. However, if there is an additional disability, a visually handicapped person *may* qualify for some of the state benefits listed below. Voluntary societies can also supplement statutory help by granting small pensions or making grants to meet specific needs, and give financial help to blind students (see page 228). The limited help available to meet travel-to-work costs is described on page 49.

Financial reliefs for the visually handicapped

Income tax relief
A blind person who pays income tax is entitled to a tax allowance of £360 (£720 if both husband and wife are blind) in addition to the normal personal allowance so the basic rate (30 per cent) tax saving can amount to £108 (or £216 if both are blind). This allowance is claimed by inserting the date of registration and the name of the registering local authority in the space provided on the income tax return form.

Rates relief
The Rating (Disabled Persons) Act 1978 entitles disabled people (this term includes the blind, and people such as the partially sighted, who

are 'substantially and permanently handicapped by illness, injury or congenital deformity') to rates relief on any part or feature of their house which is needed specifically because of their disability. This might include the central heating installed because a member of the household is blind. A garage, carport or carspace may also attract rates relief if a car is required for a blind member of the household and is 'essential or of major importance to his well-being by reason of the nature and extent of his disability'.

The amount of relief given will naturally depend on both the feature of the house for which exemption is claimed and the local level of rates. People already in receipt of supplementary benefit would gain no financial advantage from this scheme, as their rates would be covered in full by their benefit. People receiving a rates rebate are likely to gain marginally. Advice, applications forms and the leaflet *Rates Relief for Disabled Persons* can be obtained from the rates department at the local council offices (see also page 40).

National Insurance benefits

Contributory invalidity benefit (Leaflet NI 16A)
Registration as blind is not an automatic passport to invalidity benefit. This is paid, not on the basis of any specific type of illness, but on 'incapacity for work'. At first, ability to work is assessed in comparison with the person's job before the illness, but later it is compared with any job he (or she) might reasonably be expected to perform 'having regard to his age, education, experience, state of health and other personal factors'. The fact that such work may not be available is irrelevant when 'capacity for work' is assessed.

Non-contributory invalidity pension (Leaflet NI 210)
This is paid to men, single, divorced or widowed women and to married women who are separated, but receive less than £17.75 per week in maintenance, and who have not paid enough National Insurance contributions to entitle them to a contributory invalidity pension. Again, it is paid only to people who are incapable of paid work, so entitlement depends on individual circumstances and the family doctor's opinion, rather than blind registration.

Multiply handicapped school leavers aged 16 and 17 who are unable to work can count time spent claiming NCIP as part of the qualifying period for supplementary benefit long-term rate.

Housewives' non-contributory invalidity pension (Leaflet NI 214)
This is a tax-free weekly allowance of £17.75 paid to married women under 60 who have either not contributed at all, or else made insufficient contributions under the National Insurance scheme to qualify for ordinary sickness and invalidity benefit. HNCIP is paid when, due to her disability, a married woman is so incapacitated that she can neither undertake paid work not perform her normal household duties, or can only perform them with great difficulty, pain and extreme slowness. These stringent requirements have been the source of much controversy, and in 1982 the 'household duties' requirements are under review by the government.

This pension is awarded not according to the disability itself, but on the extent that the disability handicaps the applicant in her day-to-day life. It is essential, therefore, that the application form (BF 450 in leaflet NI 214 from social security offices) should be completed very carefully indeed, especially the section where various household tasks are listed. The family doctor is also required to complete a medical report which includes questions on the applicant's ability to do normal housework, so it is important that the housewife explains to him the limitations imposed by her disability.

Visually handicapped housewives suffering from an additional handicap are amongst applicants most likely to qualify, but each case is decided on its merits and blind housewives, especially those who have recently almost completely lost their sight and are finding housework exceedingly slow, and sometimes impossible, should not be deterred from applying. Advice and help in completing the claim form may be of crucial importance; social workers, especially those specialising in welfare rights, and staff at Citizens Advice Bureaux are useful sources of assistance. The Disablement Income Group, aware that it is only too easy for eligible applicants to be refused benefit in the first instance, issue a helpful leaflet *Appealing About HNCIP* and their Social Work Advisory Service is willing to answer queries.

When claiming invalidity benefits earnings up to £16.50 per week from therapeutic or rehabilitative work are allowed.

War Pensions

Delayed blindness following service in the Forces
People who have lost the sight of one eye as a result of service in Her

32

Majesty's Forces or the Civil Defence organisations and who already receive a war pension in respect of that eye, may find that this pension can be increased by up to 100 per cent if the sight of the remaining eye seriously deteriorates. Even though this happens many years after the loss of sight in the first eye and may be unconnected with the original war injury, this will not affect eligibility. St Dunstan's are willing to advise all those who think they may come into this category, and are ready to make representations on their behalf with the pensions office of the Department of Health and Social Security for increased pensions and any other allowances which may be applicable.

Special allowances

Attendance allowance (Leaflet NI 205)
This is a tax-free allowance of either £23.65 or £15.75 per week. It is payable to people severely disabled, either physically or mentally, who over the previous six months have needed and will continue to need a great deal of care. To qualify the following conditions must be satisfied:
(a)   A person must be so severely disabled physically or mentally that, by day, he requires from another person either
   (i)   frequent attention throughout the day in connection with his bodily functions;
   or
   (ii)   continual supervision throughout the day in order to avoid substantial danger to himself or others.
(b)   A person must be so severely disabled physically or mentally that, *at night*, he requires from another person either
   (i)   prolonged or repeated attention during the night in connection with bodily functions;
   or
   (ii)   continual supervision throughout the night in order to avoid substantial injury to himself or others.
If both (a) and (b) apply, the higher rate allowance is paid. If only either (a) or (b) applies, the lower rate is given.
A child (aged between 2 and 16 years) must need 'attention or supervision substantially in excess of that normally required by a child of the same age and sex' in order to qualify.
Thus, registration as blind would not automatically ensure entitle-

33

ment. Qualification is basically dependent on the amount of supervision and attention required rather than the type of disability. Visually handicapped people suffering from a severe additional physical or mental handicap are those most likely to be eligible.

Deaf-blind people, in particular, are likely to qualify for this allowance. To clarify their position, the Attendance Allowance Board has issued the following statement:

'The Board regards communication as a bodily function and the child or adult with no guiding vision and no useful hearing will usually qualify for the issue of a certificate enabling the lower rate allowance to become payable. "No guiding vision" means that the person is unable to get about in unfamiliar places without the assistance of another person, whilst "no useful hearing" may be said to exist where a person is so deaf that the residual hearing, if any, is insufficient for practical oral communication and that some other means of communication involving the help of another person is normally used.'

Leaflet NI 205 gives fuller details about the allowances, and includes a claim form. It is important when claiming to describe as fully as possible the type and frequency of help needed. The Deaf-Blind Helpers League recommend that anyone completing a claim form for a deaf-blind applicant should attach to it a copy of the Attendance Allowance Board's statement, plus a paragraph on the following lines, adapted to meet the applicant's individual needs:

'The claimant fulfils a need for day attendance as s/he has been deaf since - - - and registered blind since - - - and requires the services of a suitable guide to go farther afield than the immediate neighbourhood for business and social requirements. Contacts are required to print on the hand in block letters or use the manual alphabet to communicate. Help is required to read sighted material.'

When completed, the claim form should be returned to the local social security office. It will then be forwarded to the Attendance Allowance Unit at Blackpool who will arrange for a home medical examination by one of their doctors, before a decision as to eligibility is made.

If applicants feel their claim has been wrongly refused, they should ask for a review within three months of the decision. In 1979, 70 per cent of such reviews in England were successful. The Royal National Institute for the Blind or the Deaf-Blind Helpers League will support

34

and advise deaf-blind people. Other sources of help are Citizens Advice Bureaux and the Disablement Income Group Social Work Advisory Service.

Invalid care allowance (Leaflet NI 212)
This taxable allowance of £17.75 is linked to the attendance allowance in that it is available to people of working age who have to stay at home to care for a severely disabled relative or friend who receives the attendance allowance (at either rate) or the constant attendance allowance paid with a war pension.

Unfortunately, it is not paid to a married woman who gives up her job to care for her husband or any other relative, though her rights to her basic National Insurance pension will be protected as her record will be credited with contributions during this period.

Mobility allowance (Leaflet NI 211)
This taxable allowance of £16.50 per week is payable to people who are unable, or virtually unable, to walk and are likely to be so incapacitated for at least a year. 'Virtual inability to walk' is assessed by taking into account the distance which (or the speed at which, or the length of time for which, or the manner in which) the applicant can walk without severe discomfort. The fact that an applicant cannot walk freely because of not being able to see what is ahead is not felt to be relevant. Blind people with additional disabilities which affect mobility are likely to qualify.

Applicants must be aged at least 5, and not more than 65, years of age. Full details and a claim form are in leaflet NI 211.

Supplementary benefit
In order to qualify for consideration for supplementary benefit, a claimant must have no more than £2,000 capital. The value of a house he or his wife owns and lives in is ignored.

The amount of supplementary allowance or pension that can then be paid is determined by the size of the gap between the claimant's present income ('resources') and the level of income that the government decides is needed to live on ('requirements'). Registered blind people are considered to need £1.25 per week more than sighted people in order to meet any extra expenses incurred through their disability.

Working out 'resources'

The Supplementary Benefit Regulations determine what forms of income are taken into account in full, or how earnings are calculated and how they affect benefit.

Income taken into account in full includes all National Insurance benefits (such as retirement and invalidity pension), as well as income such as an occupational pension. The first £4 of earnings is disregarded (there is a higher disregard for single parents) and the first £4 of the wife's earnings, as is the first £4 of income from a charity. Mobility and Attendance Allowances are disregarded in full.

Working out 'requirements'

The scale rates in force in November 1981 are listed below.

	Ordinary Scale Rates	Long-term Scale Rates*
Married couple	£ 37.75	£ 47.35
Single householder *i.e. a single person directly responsible for household necessities and rent*	£ 23.25	£ 29.60
Someone aged 18 or over and living in another person's household	£ 18.60	£ 23.65
Aged 16 to 17	£ 14.30	£ 18.15
Children aged 11 to 15	£ 11.90	
under 11	£ 7.90	
Additions for claimant or dependant over age 80	£ 25p	
Blindness addition	£ 1.25	
Rent addition for non-householders	£ 2.55	

* Paid to all pensioners and those who have received supplementary benefit continuously for one year whilst not required to register for work. Disabled people working part-time and not required to register for the rest are also included, as are disabled people who only have to sign on every three months.

The sum total of the basic scale, plus the appropriate additions (see 'Additional allowances', page 37), is considered to be the amount the claimant 'requires'. When 'resources' are deducted from 'requirements' the balance represents the amount of benefit which will be paid weekly.

These rates are expected to cover normal day-to-day living expenses except rent and rates, which are worked out individually and an allowance to cover them is included in weekly benefit. There are, however, a number of extra weekly allowances which can be paid in certain circumstances in respect of heating, diet, domestic help, laundry charges and the cost of baths.

Additional allowances for claimants of supplementary benefit

Heating allowance (Leaflet SB 17): Automatic weekly allowances are made to householders whose homes are centrally heated. (£1.65 or£3.30 according to the size of their home). All householders who are 70 years of age and over, or who have a dependant of that age living with them, receive an extra £1.65 per week. A higher rate allowance (£4.05) is automatically paid to people receiving mobility or attendance allowances.

A visually handicapped person under 70 may qualify for the lower rate heating allowance if extra warmth is needed because of having:

a) chronic ill health, due for example to bronchitis, rheumatism, arthritis or anaemia or having restricted mobility due to some physical reason such as general frailty;
or b) a home difficult to heat adequately because the rooms are draughty, damp or exceptionally large.

The higher allowance is paid when:

a) extra warmth is needed because the person suffers from a physical illness or physical disability to the extent of being housebound and unable to go out alone or if there is a serious physical illness;
or b) the home is exceptionally difficult to heat adequately, for example because it is very old or in an exposed position, and the rooms are draughty, damp or exceptionally large.

Diet allowance (Leaflet SB8): An extra weekly allowance of £3.05 is paid when a special diet is needed because the claimant suffers from diabetes; a peptic, including stomach and duodenal, ulcer; a condition of the throat which causes serious difficulty in swallowing; ulcerative colitis; a form of tuberculosis for which drug treatment is being given; or from some illness which requires a diet similar to those required for the illnesses listed above. Lower rate allowances (£1.30 per week) are paid if a diet, involving extra cost, is needed in convalescence from a major illness.

Domestic help (Leaflet SB8): If the household cannot carry out their ordinary domestic tasks such as cleaning and cooking due to old age, ill health, disability or heavy family responsibilities and that help is *not* provided by a local authority (for instance, a home help), nor by a close relative who incurs only minimal expense, then the weekly amount of the charge, 'provided it is reasonable in the circumstances', will be met.

It should be noted that, apart from the three automatic heating additions first mentioned, the onus is on the visually handicapped person or a member of the household to claim these extra allowances. If health deteriorates seriously, it is especially likely that the higher rate heating allowance will be given, but it will not be received unless someone notifies the social security office – a supporting letter from the visually handicapped person's doctor is likely to help an application. Similarly, if registration changes from partially sighted to blind the blindness addition will not be received unless the social security office has been informed, preferably by the relevant local authority.

How to claim (Leaflet SB1)
The claim form in leaflet SB1, available in inkprint at post offices and in braille from the RNIB, should be sent to the nearest social security office. All claims are dealt with in confidence. Someone from the social security office will call to discuss the claim privately with the claimants in their own homes. Claimants should make sure it is known that they are registered blind, and should mention any special needs that they have. A Notice of Assessment (form A14N) will accompany the first payment of benefit, and this will explain how the allowance is calculated. Anyone who is dissatisfied can appeal against it to an independent appeals tribunal by writing to the manager of the local office within twenty-one days. There is the right to take two helpers to the hearing. A social worker, the Citizens Advice Bureau, the local Claimant's Union are all good sources of advice and help when this kind of action is being considered.

Family income supplement (Leaflet FIS 1)
This supplement is paid to anyone in full-time work who has children, but is earning a low wage – and it is for this reason that visually handicapped workers are often unfortunate enough to be eligible. A family with one child is entitled to help if the family income is below the 'qualifying level' of £74.00 per week. The supplement paid would be half the difference between the family's actual income (with child benefit and mobility and attendance allowances disregarded) and the 'qualifying level'. The 'qualifying level' rises in £8.00 steps for each additional child. A claim form and fuller details are in leaflet FIS 1.

Although the supplement itself may not be large, it has value in other respects. The family is exempted from charges for prescriptions, dental treatment and glasses under the National Health Service, and free welfare milk is available for expectant mothers and children under school age, as well as free school meals and fare refunds if any of them has to attend hospital.

Help with NHS charges

For spectacles (Leaflet M.11)
There is a charge for each lens for spectacles supplied under the National Health Service, and the cost per lens can range from £2.90 to £8.30 depending on the lens prescribed, but in certain cases where a very sophisticated lens is prescribed, the total cost including extras could be even more than this per lens. A charge is also made for National Health Service frames. Children under 16 and older children still at school are automatically exempt, as are longstay patients in hospital. People in receipt of supplementary benefit or family income supplement should tell their optician this, and sign the declaration provided, in order to be exempted.

People who have a low income should ask their optician for form F1, complete it and send it to the local social security office in the envelope provided. Fuller details are in leaflet M.11, available at post offices – it might be helpful to consult this leaflet *before* visiting the optician.

No help is available towards the cost of private lenses or private frames, although it is possible to have National Health Service lenses fitted to suitable private frames. Neither is help available to meet the cost of magnifiers purchased from a high street optician, though they can be issued on loan if prescribed through the Hospital Eye Service.

In 1975 it was announced that registered blind and partially sighted people would be exempted from charges for spectacles, but the necessary legislation is still awaited.

For prescriptions (Leaflet M.11)
Children under 16 and adults over retirement age are automatically exempt from charges, as are people receiving supplementary benefit or family income supplement. Those whose income is a little above supplementary level should complete the claim form in leaflet M.11 in order to secure exemption.

Visually handicapped people of working age may be able to secure exemption if they suffer from any of a number of 'specified conditions' including diabetes and epilepsy, or if they suffer from 'a continuing physical disability which prevents them leaving home except with the help of another person'. Fuller details are on form FP91 from the post office or social security office, which should be completed and returned to the family doctor.

Rate rebates and rent allowances
Rate rebates are available for ratepayers not receiving supplementary benefit but who have limited means, and rent rebates are available for council or New Town tenants. Rent allowances for private tenants living in either furnished or unfurnished accommodation are available as cash grants, so that the landlord is not aware of the help a tenant is receiving.

Both rebates and allowances are calculated according to scales drawn up by local authorities following guidelines laid down by the government, and each applicant's needs and resources are taken into account. Registered blind people and people registered as handicapped with their social services department (therefore, registered partially-sighted people are included) have a higher needs allowance allocated to them, which means that they receive a little more help than would a sighted person with exactly the same resources and expenses.

Further details can be found in *There's Money Off Rent* and *How to Pay Less Rates*, free leaflets obtainable from local rating departments. Application forms for these benefits are obtainable from the local housing or treasurer's department, often found at local town halls.

The Family Fund
This fund is financed by the government but is administered by the Joseph Rowntree Memorial Trust. It provides help for families caring for a severely mentally or physically handicapped child. A fit and healthy registered blind youngster might not be eligible for help, especially if there was some useful vision. But a child under 16 years of age, suffering from a severe visual handicap, especially if it was allied to an additional physical or mental handicap, would be medically eligible. The purpose of the fund is to complement the help available from other sources. Parents are asked what help they need – and one of the most common requests is for a washing machine, which can be given if the handicap causes extra laundry. There is no means test, but social and economic circumstances are taken into account. Application forms are available from the fund and after they have been completed, one of the fund's social workers will visit and discuss the application in detail.

Parents with blind or partially sighted children who are not eligible for help from the Family Fund, may well find their local voluntary society for the blind only too willing to help. For example, Derbyshire Association for the Blind purchased and loaned an electric organ to a blind child who yearned for one! Charities which exist to meet the educational needs of visually handicapped children are described on page 228.

Help from voluntary sources
There are a large number of charities which pay small pensions or make cash grants to blind people in especially difficult circumstances. A complete list appears in the RNIB publication *Directory of Agencies for the Blind* and also in *The Charities Digest*, an annual publication to be found in the reference section of public libraries. As a general rule, the majority of these charities are only able to help if they are satisfied that the applicant is receiving the full entitlement from state funds. They also want to be certain that, if a pension is granted, it will not affect the recipient's supplementary benefit.

The RNIB administers a number of charities and welcomes enquiries regarding pensions; even a small weekly pension of £1 when paid half-yearly gives pensioners a chance to buy in a stock of coal, or treat themselves to new shoes, a coat or a dress. The Institute is also always ready to consider making relatively substantial grants, perhaps in conjunction with other voluntary agencies, towards, for example, a new roof, rewiring the house, or meeting an exceptional fuel bill. All applications are considered in the context of financial need, the Institute supplying an 'assistance enquiry form' in order to establish the applicant's means. Other major charities include:

Gardner's Trust for the Blind: £15,141 was paid out in pensions in 1980/81, and grants made totalling £20,013 to various blind individuals, institutions and organisations.

London Association for the Blind: This does not limit its help to Londoners, and is exceptional in that it gives pensions and grants to registered blind and registered partially sighted people. It has over 600 pensioners and gives over £60,000 p.a. in grants and pensions.

Richmond Charitable Trust: Makes grants in cash or in kind to needy deaf/blind people to provide help which cannot be given by state welfare services.

Telephones for the Blind Fund: This will give substantial help towards the cost of installation and rental of telephones for blind people of limited means whose local authority has refused to give help under the Chronically Sick and Disabled Persons Act (see page 22), provided that they live alone, or are often alone particularly at night, or live with a partner who is also disabled by infirmity or age.

People in real need of help can approach a charity direct but it is perhaps better to consult a social worker, who can do it on their behalf. In any case, most charities send the application forms to the local authority or voluntary society, so that a social worker can complete them. Sometimes a social worker will be able to suggest a local charity which might be prepared to help. Many people, particularly older ones, are naturally shy and reluctant to ask for help, but if they can only do so they will be pleasantly surprised to find how much generosity and kindly goodwill there is around.

Getting information

The details given in this chapter are correct at the time of going to press, but there is always a possibility that they will be changed by new regulations. It is always wise to check the current position by obtaining the leaflet listed alongside each benefit, which gives more detailed information than has been possible here. These can be obtained from local social security offices (listed in telephone directories under 'H' for [Department of] Health and Social Security) or direct from the DHSS Leaflets Unit. A comprehensive leaflet *Social Security Rates* (NI 196) lists all standard rates of social security benefits, and is available at all post offices and in braille from the Royal National Institute for the Blind. *Which Benefit? 60 ways to get cash help*, an inkprint booklet issued free by the Department of Health and Social Security, is available free in braille in one volume from the Royal National Institute for the Blind.

The *Disability Rights Handbook* is published annually in November and is a comprehensive guide to income benefits, aids and services for handicapped people. It can be ordered from the Disability Alliance. The Disablement Income Group publishes a series of short, straightforward guides to the major benefits under the title *A Guide to Help you Overcome some Hurdles*. Topics covered include sickness and invalidity benefit, non-contributory invalidity pension, housewife's non-contributory invalidity benefit, attendance allowance, invalid care allowance and mobility allowance. The booklets give advice on how to complete the necessary forms and also answer the questions that are most often asked about each benefit. They can be obtained direct from the Disablement Income Group in inkprint.

Don't forget your smile when you go out. You get much more help that way!
(Peter White)

4 Employment

Like those for the rest of the general public, employment services for the visually handicapped are provided through the Manpower Services Commission; for people with severe visual defects these services are linked with and reinforced by voluntary societies. All registered blind and partially sighted people available for work may, if they wish, be registered as disabled with the Commission. This makes them eligible for the special facilities described in this chapter, and also gives them some advantage in finding work as employers with an average work-force of twenty or more are required to employ a 3 per cent quota of disabled people. Failure to employ the full quota is not an offence, but, if a firm so fails, it is subject to the following restrictions:

a) it must not engage staff other than those registered as disabled unless specially exempted, *and*

b) it must not discharge a registered disabled employee without sufficient cause. This also applies if the discharge would bring the firm below its quota.

Failure to comply with either of these provisions *is* an offence.

The Disabled Persons Register

The Register is kept in two main sections:

i) for people capable of ordinary employment

ii) for the severely disabled who need special working conditions.

There are two further subdivisions for the visually handicapped:

i) for registered blind and those partially-sighted people whose BD8s indicate that they would benefit from 'training for employment or other services appropriate to the blind'

ii) for those with eye defects (which includes the rest of the partially sighted register).

The Manpower Services Commission works through its two executive divisions, the Employment Service Division (ESD) and the Training Service Division (TSD). Information about these agencies and advice on registering as disabled can be obtained from local Jobcentres or employment offices.

Employment Service Division
The agency provides a resettlement service through its Blind Persons'

Resettlement Officers (BPROs) for those who are registered blind and for partially sighted people who would benefit from training for employment by blind methods. Other partially sighted jobseekers who wish to get in touch with the Resettlement Service should do so by contacting their local Disablement Resettlement Officer (DRO), again through a Jobcentre or employment exchange.

There are, however, only thirty-six BPROs in the entire country and, as the nature of their work takes them away from their main office for much of the time, they tend to be elusive. The local Jobcentre or employment office can always act as a channel of communication between jobseeker and BPRO and the BPRO can always be asked to go and visit the jobseeker at home. In an attempt to provide a more local service in one area the duties of BPROs and DROs have been combined, but results of this experiment are, as yet, inconclusive. In England and Wales the RNIB work closely with the BPROs in finding jobs in the commercial and professional fields.

Referral to the BPRO should be done automatically by the local authority when a client who is available for work is registered blind or partially sighted. However, there is no reason why newly registered people should not set the wheels in motion themselves by notifying their local Jobcentre of their handicap, or approaching the RNIB Employment and Assistance Department direct. In many cases it would be wise to do so.

Employment rehabilitation courses: The BPRO can arrange courses at the RNIB Employment Rehabilitation Centre at Torquay, or at Alwyn House, Ceres, Fife. Both centres aim to help men and women of working age to adjust to visual handicap and to regain their confidence in everyday activities. In addition, skills and abilities are assessed and realistic vocational guidance given. Braille, typing and mobility are taught, whilst woodwork, pottery and other craft classes aim to increase manual dexterity. In the assembly and machine shops residents are assessed for their suitability for further training in light engineering or for direct entry into industry. At Torquay instruction in the long-cane technique is available, and there is considerable emphasis on the use of residual vision. The provision of low vision aids is discussed with those who would benefit by them, and advice is given as to their correct use.

The courses vary between four and twelve weeks according to individual needs and in exceptional cases can be extended to twenty-

45

six weeks. All fees are paid by the ESD, and residents receive a tax-free maintenance allowance at a higher rate than basic unemployment or sickness benefit. Free travel warrants to and from the centres are issued.

Towards the end of the course, the resident joins in discussions regarding the future, and finally a recommendation is made for further training or for placement in a job. In some cases this will mean that the visually handicapped person returns to his or her previous employment, having gained enough self-confidence to tackle the old job again. Others will go direct into industry.

The Training Services Division

The majority of people completing a rehabilitation course are recommended for a further specific training course. These are offered through the Training Opportunities Scheme (TOPS) provided both by the TSD itself, and through its sponsorship of trainees on courses run by voluntary agencies. All TOPS courses are free, and in addition, trainees receive a weekly tax-free allowance. All courses listed below are available to registered blind people and partially sighted people who would benefit by training by blind methods, and, where indicated, to those 'with eye defects' (see page 44).

Light engineering: The TSD Skillcentre (Pixmore Avenue, Letchworth, Hertfordshire SG14 1PU; tel. 046 26 3084) provides an eight-week introductory course. Assembly, inspection work, and machine operating using vertical and horizontal mills and drilling machines are included, but the major part of trainees' time is spent in learning to operate a wide range of capstan lathes. When employment has been obtained, further 'on the job' training can be given by the BPTO (see page 49). The length and content of the residential course can be varied to meet individual requirements. It is designed to meet the needs of blind and all categories of partially sighted people.

The Queen Alexandra College, Birmingham, offers a two-year engineering training programme, designed primarily but not exclusively for school leavers. The course includes attendance one day a week at Warley College of Technology and successful students can obtain a Union of Education Institute certificate. A vocational course in bicycle repairs, a new field for the visually handicapped, is also offered.

Shorthand and audio typing: A one-year shorthand typing and/or a two-term audio typing course is offered by the RNIB Commercial College in London. The courses are residential and students are expected to reach a shorthand speed of 100 words per minute and to pass the RSA Intermediate Typing examination.

Telephony: The RNIB Commercial College offers a six-week residential course giving instruction in the operation of a range of private board exchanges. Alternatively, it is sometimes possible for the RNIB to provide 'on the job' training for visually handicapped people who have obtained employment as switchboard operators.

These three commercial courses are all intensive. Students require a good basic knowledge of typing and a reasonable standard of braille before they start; or, in the case of would-be telephonists, ability to read and write using low vision aids. The RNIB selection board looks for candidates who have not only aptitude and potential, but also a high degree of mobility and independence. The majority of students are under fifty years of age. However, in 1981 the content and scope of these courses is under review and the RNIB is considering a recommendation made in *The Employment of Blind People* (the report of a working party, published by the RNIB in 1979) that a purpose-built or specially adapted commercial college should be provided, closely related to an establishment offering commercial education to sighted students.

Commercial courses for school-leavers: Courses are available at Queen Alexandra College, Birmingham and the Royal National College, Hereford (p. 226–7).

Computer programming: Nine-week courses are held at the RNIB Commercial College. A good educational background is required and candidates need to have numerate and logical minds. Good communication skills achieved either through efficient braille and typing or by the competent use of low vision aids are essential.

Optacon reading: Following an aptitude test, the RNIB Commercial College offers basic training in the Optacon for people already in employment whose career prospects would be improved by the acquisition of this skill. Courses last for two weeks, but can be extended to three or four weeks. Average speeds of reading achieved are twenty to thirty words per minute. (See also p. 148.)

Craftwork: Training in a wide range of crafts, including chair caning, rush seating, brush-making, basketry and wrought iron work is offered to potential home-workers (see page 51) by the *RNIB Home Industries Department, 2 Alma Road, Reigate, Surrey RH2 0AS Reigate (tel: 073 72 44701)* and at the Queen Alexandra College, Birmingham.

Piano Tuning: This well-established trade for blind people has in recent years enjoyed an increase in popularity, and job opportunities on successfully completing training are good.

Non-residential courses lasting seven terms are offered to registered blind people and all classes of partially sighted people at the *London College of Furniture, 41 Commercial Road, London E1 (tel. 01-247 1953)*. The Royal National College for the Blind, Hereford, offers a three-year residential course. Selection boards look for a good sense of pitch and good hearing within the normal audiometric range. Good mobility and a pleasant personality are also important attributes.

Physiotherapy: A full-time three-year residential course is available at the *RNIB North London School of Physiotherapy, 10 Highgate Hill, Archway, London N19 5ND (tel. 01-272 1659)* leading to the certificate of the Chartered Society of Physiotherapists, holders of which are eligible for state registration.

Candidates should normally be between 18 and 35 years of age and physically fit and healthy as the work is strenuous. School leavers are required to have five GCE passes at 'O' level including one science subject, and one pass at 'A' level. These requirements can be modified for mature students with relevant experience. A reasonable standard of braille and typing is needed, together with good mobility and an ability to get on well with people. The selection procedure includes a stay of a week in the school. Initial acceptance for training is for a six-month probationary period.

Professional careers
Apart from physiotherapy there are no special training schemes for the visually handicapped. However, many visually handicapped peo-

ple qualify as teachers, solicitors, musicians, and social workers following the same courses as sighted students. Where local education authority grants are not available, the TSD Professional Training Scheme will help blind adults to undertake a vocational course, including university degree courses, with the object of providing an adequate livelihood. Advice and guidance regarding this scheme and the facilities available for blind students is available from the BPRO and the RNIB Education Department respectively.

Training and employment for ex-service and semi-service personnel
The Gubbay Trust, set up by St Dunstan's, offers training, settlement in a job and aftercare to ex-service men under 50 years of age, whose blindness is *not* attributable to war service. In addition, members of uniformed organisations, such as the police, firemen, and so on who have lost their sight on duty are also eligible for similar help. Full details are available from St Dunstan's.

Help on the job

Blind Persons' Training Officers (BPTOs)
The Employment Service Division (ESD) has eleven specialist staff with this title. They are responsible for special training on the job and advise on technical matters such as the adaptation of machines. The BPTO may accompany workers in the first few days of employment to help them find their way around the factory as well as to and from work. This advice and help is available to both employer and employee throughout the visually handicapped person's working life. The RNIB offers a similar service to people in commercial or professional occupations in England and Wales.

'Fares to work' scheme
The ESD has power to give financial help when visually handicapped workers are unable to use public transport to reach their place of employment. This may be because they suffer from an additional disability or because public transport does not exist. In such cases, the cost of a taxi can be met, either for the whole journey or to the nearest source of public transport. Leaflet DPL 13, obtainable at Jobcentres, gives details, and requests are handled through the local DRO and BPRO.

Aids to employment
Aids which are essential if a visually handicapped person is to be able
to work efficiently, or which it can be shown would increase the
capacity to work, can be borrowed from the ESD. These include
items such as braille micrometers, pocket memo tape recorders,
braille machines, typewriters, industrial magnifiers and the very
expensive talking calculators and closed-circuit television sets. Low
vision aids, including CCTV, are supplied only after a full low vision
assessment either at Moorfields Hospital (London), Aston University
(Birmingham), or Glasgow Institute of Technology. Every application is considered on an individual basis, and visually handicapped
people should contact their BPRO or the RNIB Employment Officer.

Personal reading service
The Manpower Services Commission has accepted in principle the
provision of a grant-aided reading service aimed at assisting blind
people employed in commercial, clerical and professional occupations
to overcome the problems created by the need to use written material
in their work. In 1982 the scheme has yet to be implemented.

Sheltered employment
This term describes working conditions that are specially designed to
meet the needs of visually handicapped or disabled workers. Tradi-
tionally, sheltered employment has been the preserve of blind people
who could not meet the demands of open industry, but were competent in the craft skills of willow-work, brush- and mat-making.
Nowadays, special factories (sheltered workshops) increasingly concentrate on wirework, light engineering, plastics, furniture-making,
packing and assembly work, whilst the 'home-worker schemes'
include music teachers, shopkeepers, radio repairers and carpenters
as well as basket-makers and piano tuners.

Admission to sheltered employment
This is a matter of agreement between the voluntary association or
local authority running the scheme, and the ESD (represented by the
BPRO). Because of the economic recession, if all other job prospects
are very bleak, BPROs may well recommend for sheltered employment job seekers classed as suitable for open industry. At a time of 'nil
growth' however, local authorities running schemes may well be

reluctant to accept new entrants. The National League of the Blind and Disabled are always ready to advise applicants and, where necessary, help them press their case with the appropriate authorities.

Home-worker schemes are run by local authorities (social services departments) or by voluntary agencies. They help not only blind people who have additional handicaps and could not work in open industry, or who live in isolated parts of the country, but also those who have the skills and qualities needed to develop successful businesses and who have the potential for becoming independent, self-employed people. To be included in the scheme, a worker must reach the minimum earning rate for the relevant trade. Earnings are then augmented on a sliding scale by the local authority. As the earnings of the worker increase, so the augmentation decreases, and ceases when earnings approximately reach the basic wage which would be received in a sheltered workshop. Both the minimum earning rates and augmentation scale rates are regularly reviewed by the Local Authorities Advisory Committee on the Conditions of Service for Blind People.

Home-workers are self-employed, but receive supervision and support from the administering agency. This includes the provision of tools, equipment and a workshop, the purchase of materials and marketing of produce if needed, and technical and business advice. Home-worker schemes are unevenly distributed over the country; the majority are found in the south.

Sheltered workshops are also run by local authorities or voluntary agencies. Prospective employees need to be reasonably independent and mobile and there is no formal age limit, but retirement age is normally 65 years. A few workshops have hostel accommodation. All workers must be able to meet minimum productivity levels. Conditions of employment, including the basic wage rate which compares favourably with the rate in ordinary factories, are determined by the National Association of Industries for the Blind and Disabled, a body which represents both employers and workers.

This chapter has concentrated on the traditional work that has been done, in some cases for many years, by blind people, for it is primarily in these areas that special training and facilities are available. But blind people hold down jobs in a much wider variety of fields. In

51

offices, there are blind managers, executives, sales representatives; in the country, one can find blind farmers, market gardeners and poultry keepers. On *In Touch* we have had interviews with a motor mechanic, a publican, a museum curator, a book wholesaler and a food taster, to name but a few.

Nevertheless, finding a job is one of the most difficult problems being faced by anyone whose sight has recently been lost. Especially disturbing are the declining prospects for blind people as manual workers in industry. The steady decrease in the percentage of blind people finding work as machine operators in the engineering industry is an unhappy example. The appointment by the RNIB in 1980 of a research officer, part of whose brief is work on the development of new employment opportunities, may indicate better times ahead. Another encouraging aspect is the proportional increase in the number of blind people in 'white collar' jobs. Office work, return to which seems out of the question when lying in hospital, may be possible thanks to modern technology and low vision aids. It is more than ever essential for employer and employee to check with the professionals before labelling a job 'impossible'. RNIB Employment Officers, based in Bristol, Birmingham, Merseyside, Newcastle-on-Tyne and the Midlands are always available for consultation and can be easily contacted through the RNIB London office.

It would be wrong, however, to end this chapter giving the impression that aids, training and services alone are sufficient to solve an employment problem. The determination and drive of the blind person counts for far more.

'I made no move to leave,' said John White, a cabin cleaner for British Gypsum, referring to the time he lost his sight.

'You've got to shine in some other way,' was the comment of Harry Foster, a registered blind hospital porter.

It is not unusual for blind people to find themselves work when all the 'helping agencies' have failed. No one denies that it is a battle to find a job, but it is one that is won by over 700 blind people every year.

Further reading
Looking for Jobs: An Introduction to the Rights of Blind and Partially Sighted People. National Federation of the Blind of the UK. Braille and inkprint. 59 Silversea Drive, Westcliff-on-Sea, Essex SSO 9XD

(Southend (0702) 74059). Includes addresses of all sheltered work-shops.

Blind People at Work and *Looking for Work*. Free leaflets from the RNIB.

Employment and Careers. Section 0.8 Information Sheets. The Partially Sighted Society. 1980. Includes names and addresses of all BPRO's, and BPTO's and RNIB Employment Officers.

Aids and Adaptations for Disabled Employees. Leaflet EPL 71. Free from Jobcentres.

A list of cassette tapes describing employment opportunities for visually handicapped people in a wide range of jobs can be obtained from the RNIB Employment Section.

★ *The easiest way to find your coat when its hung up with many others in a cloakroom is to turn one sleeve inside out, or if you don't want to be that conspicuous, put a safety pin just inside the cuff.*
(David Scott Blackhall)

★ *I frequently drop my self-threading needle or put it down and forget where. Now I keep a large magnet handy. This I draw across my clothing and over the carpet around me, and come up with the needle in seconds.*
(Mrs. I. Knight, Ruislip)

5 Housing and homes

As 75 per cent of people with very poor sight are over retirement age, one principal question to be faced is often: 'Can I manage on my own?' There may also be a nagging doubt: 'Should I go into a home?' This chapter describes the services people can expect to find to help them live in their own homes and sets out the possible alternatives.

All social workers aim to help their elderly clients live as independently as possible for as long as possible. If someone has just been registered as blind, no official is automatically going to think that he or she is no longer fit to live alone. This is more likely to be the reaction of relatives and friends. One of the golden rules for anyone with poor sight, living alone, is not to rush into any hasty decisions about the future. Time is needed to adjust, and relatives and friends also need to give themselves time to come to terms with the new situation. This is discussed further in Chapter 18.

Living independently

Help in the home
Running a home can be very hard work, especially for older people. In addition, people with poor sight have to concentrate extra hard all the time, which is in itself very tiring.

The home help service, supplied through all local authorities, brings a willing pair of hands into the home – and these are worth more than any gadget. If someone is finding housework increasingly difficult, the doctor, health visitor or social worker can refer him or her to social services for this help. How much is given depends on the need and the number of home helps available. The average is two visits each week of between two and two and a half hours – long enough to cope with basic jobs such as cleaning the kitchen and bathroom.

Home helps often will do some shopping, wash the 'smalls' or prepare a simple meal. Generally, the rules do not allow them to do heavy jobs such as spring-cleaning. On the other hand, the home help often becomes a real friend and does far more than she is required to do in the course of her duty. Payment for this service varies from one local authority to another. Sometimes it is assessed according to the householder's means, sometimes there is a flat-rate charge, sometimes there is no charge at all. This last variation is becoming increasingly rare in 1982 as financial cutbacks take effect. No money is paid directly to the home help. Those who receive the service are sent an account regularly, and the amount paid is known only to them and the authority concerned.

Meals

Preparing meals and shopping for food can be a real nightmare when poor sight and indifferent health go together. In most areas, a meals-on-wheels service operates to bring a hot dinner to the home generally twice a week, or, in some areas, every weekday. The cost of the meals is modest, generally being subsidised. Another solution is to join a day centre or luncheon club. A number of voluntary societies and local authorities run such centres, where a hot midday meal is provided. In addition, of course, there is the chance to chat with other people and to benefit from the chiropody, hairdressing and social activities that are often also provided. Some centres have various food products for sale at reduced prices, such as Bovril, Complan, Marmite, Ribena. Transport may be provided for people who cannot reach the centre without it. The social worker or health visitor can explain what facilities there are in each district.

Home improvements

People in old houses which, although soundly built, lack modern amenities, can apply for a grant from the local council to help modernise them. Intermediate grants can cover half the cost of any missing standard amenity (bath or shower, washbasin, kitchen sink, hot and cold water supply, indoor WC) or provide an alternative standard amenity when the existing one, such as an upstairs toilet, is inaccessible due to the disabled person's handicap. Improvement grants (between half and three quarters of the cost depending where the applicant lives) can cover work which needs to be done to make the home suitable for a disabled person to live or work in. Applicants may get help to meet their share of the cost from social services, under Section 2 of the Chronically Sick and Disabled Persons Act if the department is satisfied that the alteration is essential.

The provisions for these grants are complicated, but full details are available at local council offices; or the Citizens Advice Bureau would always be ready to advise.

Home insulation: Households where the loft and hot and cold water tanks are not insulated can receive a grant from their local council of 66 per cent (maximum £65) towards the cost of insulation materials. For people in 'special need' (which means elderly people receiving supplementary benefit, rates rebate or rent allowances) a higher grant rate of 90 per cent or £90, whichever is the least, applies.

Work must not be started until the council has approved the application, but people in 'special need' have priority on the waiting list. Full details and application forms are obtainable at local council offices.

Safety

To an outsider, elderly peoples' homes may seem full of hazards but, even though people are visually handicapped, if they are familiar with every awkward step and every piece of furniture, they may in fact be far safer and healthier in their own home than if moved to a modern, uncluttered, centrally heated environment. A room may be so filled with furniture that it enables someone who is unsteady to get about safely, as everything is within grabbing distance. To tidy the room and provide a walking frame may well cause problems rather than solve them.

The bathroom and kitchen are, of course, rooms where accidents are liable to occur. Again, the decision to make alterations has to be weighed against the risks caused just by making those alterations.

A bath mat for inside the bath is nearly always welcomed, and most elderly visually handicapped people would appreciate a grab rail – if it could be fitted where *they* think it is necessary. And this can only be decided by a 'dry-run' – many a grab rail ends up as a home for the flannel as it has been placed according to the fitter's armlength, rather than the user's! And it is equally important to consider the feelings and attitudes of the visually handicapped themselves. A new 'click' ignition lighter (see page 68) for the ancient gas stove, to be used instead of matches, might well be acceptable – suggestions to replace the actual stove with a small electric cooker might not be. The user needs the reassurance of old, remembered things. (Safety in regard to stairs is considered on page 122.)

Gas safety: British Gas make no charge for checking gas appliances of blind or handicapped people (including the partially sighted) who live alone. Necessary adjustments are made and minor parts costing under

£2.50 (plus VAT) are replaced free. Where more expensive repair work is needed, a written estimate is sent, as help with this is sometimes possible through social security or social services. Meters can be moved to a more accessible position for a standard charge of £3, though the cost would be more if the distance involved exceeded three ·feet. A free, easy-to-use, handle can be fitted to a pre-payment meter for people finding the coin mechanism difficult to operate; or if they decide instead to have a credit meter, no charge will be made for the change.

Requests for this service must be through social services departments or voluntary societies. A large-print leaflet 'Free Gas Safety Checks for Elderly and Disabled Customers' explains the scheme fully and should be found in local showrooms.

Calling for help
Social services or the local voluntary society may be able to help with this problem – certainly with advice, perhaps by putting the blind person in touch with a neighbourhood help scheme, or by installing appropriate equipment. This can range from a simple card to place in the window to the most sophisticated electronic aid which, when a small body-worn radio transmitter is pressed, automatically dials a pre-set sequence of telephone numbers until one is answered, when it delivers a pre-recorded message asking for help. Current details of the many different emergency call systems can be obtained from the Disabled Living Foundation.

When isolation is a very acute problem, the local authority may be able to help with the cost of installing and renting a telephone. The circumstances in which this help is given are described on page 22. If the local authority cannot help, the Telephones for the Blind Fund may assist (page 42). Some voluntary societies for the blind also help – for example, Cornwall County Association for the Blind spent nearly £6,000 in 1975/76 on telephones for blind people in Cornwall.

Nursing services at home
The home nursing service is well known, and the community nurse is a very familiar friend to many blind people. Some areas, in addition, provide a night nursing service for elderly people who are gravely ill. Incontinence can be a heart-breaking problem, but there is a variety of aids available nowadays, through the community nurse or health visitor, which should help overcome this. The Disabled Living

Foundation can also give practical advice on this problem. Some local authorities provide a laundry service, some provide home nursing aids, such as special beds, commodes, bed cradles and aids to prevent pressure sores. Who supplies what varies in different parts of the country, but the patient's doctor, nurse, health visitor or social worker should be able to pinpoint the local source of supply.

Chapter 18, *Help for the very elderly*, gives more information specifically related to the needs of old people.

Sheltered housing

Sometimes the problems of continuing to live alone seem insuperable. The house may be too large, too isolated and too inconvenient, and the garden a constant source of anxiety. An elderly person may be marooned in a top flat, with stairs too steep and difficult to climb. This may seem to be the time to consider alternative accommodation.

Local authority housing

Nowadays local authorities provide a variety of housing for elderly people living in unsuitable accommodation. Flats and bungalows are designed for easy running, and, in the newer developments, central heating is usual. Sheltered housing, a group of flats or bungalows linked to a warden's house by an alarm system and intercom, are increasingly common. Each flat or bungalow usually consists of a bedroom, lounge (or bed-sitting room), kitchen and bathroom. There is usually also a large communal lounge, where residents can meet; and often a laundry room is provided. Occasionally there is a communal dining room as well, where a midday meal can be enjoyed if desired, or this facility may be provided at a nearby old people's home.

Rents for this type of accommodation are generally reasonable and within the rent allowance paid by the Supplementary Benefits Commission, so that people eligible for a supplementary pension need not worry. People not eligible for supplementary pension may of course qualify for a rent rebate (see page 40).

Applicants have to satisfy the local housing department that they have lived in the area for a number of years, and to complete an application form containing questions about their present accommodation; the more unsuitable it is, the greater the priority on the waiting list. A medical certificate from the doctor and a supporting letter from a social worker will help. But the waiting lists are always long and, in practice, vacancies generally go to council tenants living in houses too large for them; though some housing departments will consider applications from handicapped owner-occupiers who are willing to sell their home to the department at an agreed price in return for more suitable council accommodation. Housing schemes are also run by voluntary housing associations and private charities; and applicants who live in their own homes or in privately rented accommodation would probably stand a better chance of being rehoused by applying to one of these.

Voluntary housing associations
A limited amount of housing is provided by voluntary housing associations for blind and partially-sighted people whose sight is likely to deteriorate. The trustees of the Gift of Thomas Pocklington administer three schemes. Pocklington Court, Roehampton, provides both single and double flats. Pocklington Place, Birmingham and Pocklington Rise, Plymouth both provide single and double flats, together with meals and warden supervision if this is needed, and both are linked to fully residential homes with nursing wings. Applicants for these flats, which are all purpose-built to a very high standard, should be retired and capable of looking after themselves.

The London Association for the Blind also has private flats in South and Central London and fifty-eight flats in Epsom for single blind people, and for married couples where at least one partner is blind or partially sighted. The Association will consider applications from any part of the country. The Star Housing Assocation has five flats in Acton in a converted house, and at Colindale in North London it has a housing project consisting of twelve single and double flatlets, six bungalows and eight family houses. Other voluntary societies for the blind in Blackpool, Croydon, Ipswich, Norwich, Walsall, Worthing and Leicester have similar schemes.

Residential homes
Every local authority has to provide residential accommodation for people 'who by reason of age, infirmity, or any other circumstance are in need of care and attention which is not otherwise available to them'. This may be in large, old-fashioned buildings which still, despite efforts to make them bright and attractive inside, retain an institu-

tional air. More often, however, private houses have been modernised and adapted, or new premises built. There may be no steps, but grab rails along all corridors, electric lifts, a very high standard of furnishing and a reasonable proportion of single rooms, and many blind people find that their needs are well met by the facilities offered in such a purpose-built home, and that they can live a fuller life in a community where the majority of residents are sighted, although very frail and handicapped. Some local authorities have, in addition, special homes for the blind – of course, some blind people prefer a specialist home.

Waiting lists for local authority homes tend to be long, though admission is always to the applicant in greatest need at the time a vacancy occurs. Someone with limited means would have greater priority than someone with financial reserves adequate to pay for any suitable private accommodation that might be available. The local social services department can provide a list of private accommodation (often known as 'rest homes') for elderly people in their area, as all such homes have to be registered with them. In addition, in some areas there is a 'boarding-out scheme', where the local authority will try to put an elderly person in touch with a family prepared to have him or her as a paying guest.

Many local voluntary societies for the blind have their own specialist homes, and are increasingly offering vacancies to visually handicapped people living outside their areas. Some major agencies also consider applications from blind people irrespective of where they live. Amongst these are the Royal National Institute for the Blind who can supply a free brochure giving details of their homes in Westgate-on-Sea in Kent, Harrogate in Yorkshire and in Hove, Sussex (the last for women only), and special homes for the deaf-blind at Harrogate and Burnham-on-Sea; the Gift of Thomas Pocklington with three purpose-built homes, in Birmingham, Plymouth and Northwood; the London Association for the Blind with homes in Horley, Surrey and in South Croydon and North London Homes for the Blind with three homes on the Sussex coast for middle-aged and elderly people.

A list of homes for adult blind people is issued by the RNIB and also appears in the *Directory of Agencies for the Blind*. Accommodation for younger, multiply handicapped blind people is discussed on page 257.

Finances

In all local authority homes, payment is on a sliding scale. Those unable to meet the full charge (often about £80 per week) are asked to complete a financial statement, and then assessed to pay a proportion of the charge according to their means. It is always assumed that a person must have an income of £5.90 per week (uprated annually) left for pocket money. This means that, for someone whose only income is the retirement pension and whose capital is very limited, the weekly charge would be £23.70. The difference between that and the full charge is met by the local authority. The greater a person's capital or income, the higher the charge; but, as capital or income decreases, so the contribution towards the fees is also reduced.

Most voluntary homes have a similar scheme for the payment of fees, as they have generally entered into an agreement with the local authority which has approved the 'full charge', and agreed to subsidise residents. However, because of the economic situation, it cannot be taken for granted that all local authorities are willing to do this.

Even when a person has elected to pay the full charge (which may be a very reasonable one), the voluntary society may still ask the local authority to act as a sponsor in case financial help is needed at a later date, though, depending on the circumstances, they may not insist on this sponsorship.

It is certainly a good idea for any blind person to talk the whole matter over with a social worker. She can help to complete the necessary forms, and also answer detailed questions about local homes, and possibly arrange visits. Sometimes a would-be resident can have a 'holiday' fortnight, either to get a break from housekeeping, or to enable relatives to go on holiday. This is an ideal way for elderly people to find out just how well they would settle into community life.

Fees charged by private homes ('rest homes') as described on page 60 can be met through supplementary benefit. Local authorities, through their social services departments, have the power (but not the duty) to 'top up' these allowances. This power is not often exercised at present.

Private nursing homes and residential homes are expensive, but it is not always realised that residents may be eligible for supplementary benefit if they no longer own any property, have not more than £2,000 capital and limited income – though the first £4 per week of annuity, trust income or war disablement pension is ignored, as are attendance and mobility allowances (see page 33–35). This state retirement pension is of course taken into account in full. This supplementary allowance is statutory and is composed of four elements: board/lodging, an extra board/lodging allowance for long-term boarders over pension age, and a personal expenses allowance.

In London and the Home Counties, where rates are a little higher, this allowance could total £75.80, whilst registered blind people would also receive an extra £1.25 and, if they received attendance and mobility allowances, an extra £4.05 heating addition as well. If there is still a difference between the resident's supplemented income and the fees, this can be met by a relative or a charity without affecting the supplementary benefit paid. Counsel and Care for the Elderly issue a useful free fact sheet giving full details of the current rates and how to claim benefit.

Nursing care

Most of the homes mentioned so far expect their new residents to be reasonably mobile, and to be able to wash and dress themselves. This is, perhaps, especially true of voluntary homes and private rest homes, where an age limit for admission may well have been decided. Over recent years, however, the average age of new residents has risen steadily, and all homes have had to adapt themselves to the needs of older, frailer residents; but for someone in need of nursing care, or who is incontinent, the problem of accommodation can be very difficult.

Some local authorities have homes for people who need extra care, or who are mentally confused, but demand for these places always exceeds supply. Few blind homes can offer nursing care, though Pocklington Court, Northwood, caters for elderly frail visually handicapped people. Essex Voluntary Association for the Blind is unique in having a nursing home at Frinton-on-Sea for registered blind, partially sighted or handicapped people. Permanent residents, convalescent and holiday guests are welcomed from any part of the country.

Nursing homes in general would, of course, rarely reject an applicant on grounds of blindness. The Area Health Authority keeps a register of all nursing homes (which differ mainly from the private 'rest homes' mentioned in that they must have a trained nurse on their staff, and on duty day and night). Another source of information is Counsel and Care for the Elderly (the Elderly Invalids Fund) a national charity which offers advice on all matters concerning retired people, including accommodation. The Fund visits homes in Greater London annually and gives sources of information on homes in other parts of the country. The best local people to approach for advice are the patient's doctor or health visitor. They will know local nursing homes and also be able to discuss whether admission to a short- or a long-stay bed in the geriatric department of the local hospital is either an appropriate or possible alternative.

A blind friend, who is over eighty and lives alone, has the following arrangement with his next-door-neighbour. The neighbour has her morning newspaper delivered to my blind friend who then puts the newspaper in the neighbour's letterbox. If the newspaper is not put in then the neighbour would instantly know that something was wrong. Quite a good idea for keeping in touch with a minimum of trouble to both parties.
(James Grady, Dundee)

As I am totally blind and live alone I cannot tell whether any letters have been delivered. They used to lie on the mat for days until a visitor called. Then I had the idea of suspending a small cow bell behind the letter box so that any time something is delivered I hear the bell jingle!
(Margaret Huscroft, Walton-on-Thames)

6 Everyday living

Many blind people, given time and practice, learn to manage most ordinary household tasks. Memory, tidiness and an increasing awareness of the information that can be conveyed by the other senses all play their part in this. This chapter can only give outline guidance on how blind people manage, but it may serve to start people thinking on how they can solve their particular problem.

Looking after yourself

Clothes
Blind people usually have no difficulty in dressing themselves, but they may find it difficult to distinguish similar garments of different colours. It is possible to get from the RNIB a set of special buttons in which each of eight colours is represented by an easily identifiable shape (e.g. red is represented by a cross, green by a shamrock and blue by a star). The buttons can be sewn, pinned or glued on to clothes and can withstand machine-washing or dry-cleaning. A set of twenty assorted 'Shapes for colour' buttons costs 69p (concession price). People who can read some braille might like to use woven braille tapes which are available in fourteen different colours. It is also possible to get labels with the alphabet in braille and the manufacturers are prepared to weave personal names or any other special requirement in braille. Details from *J & J Cash Ltd, Kingfield Road, Coventry, CV1 4DU (tel: Coventry (0203) 555222)*.

But even without such labels it is possible, with experience, to distinguish a green jacket from a brown one by the difference in texture of material, or by noticing that one has fewer buttons on the sleeve. Perhaps the simplest way is always to keep an object such as a handkerchief or a pencil in the breast pocket of one particular jacket. Many blind men hang matching ties together with their suits or jackets and keep brown and black shoes firmly apart. Some men always tie the laces together after taking off their shoes to keep the pairs together; another simple trick is to put a tiny piece of sticking plaster inside the heels of a brown pair of shoes to distinguish them from the black. Pairing socks and stockings presents some difficulty; to avoid this, some people buy all their footwear in one colour.

It is probably easier for a woman to distinguish her dresses, as these come in a wide variety of styles and materials; it is again useful to try and remember some easily felt characteristics – or to create one, for example, by always keeping a brooch pinned on to the green dress. Matching belts should always be kept with the dress; matching gloves put inside the appropriate handbag. As with other aspects of coping with blindness, a good memory and tidy habits make life much easier. Some elderly people with little or no sight find it very difficult to cope with ordinary clothes fastenings such as zips, hooks or buttons. There are a few manufacturers who specialise in making clothes with easy-to-use fastenings for men and women. Details are available from the Disabled Living Foundation's information service.

Obviously colours are a matter of individual taste, and a good friend who will honestly say what suits a blind person is the best, positive help. It might also be worth remembering, in the interests of safety, that a light coloured top-coat will help motorists to see a blind pedestrian. On a grey, rainy day it is not easy for a motorist to see a pedestrian dressed in dark colours. For extra protection, it is possible to buy from the Royal Society for the Prevention of Accidents orange arm bands incorporating a grey reflective strip. The bright orange colour can be seen easily on a dull day when there is no lighting; the grey reflective strip picks up the lights of approaching cars. A pair of armbands costs 47p (including VAT) and can be obtained from *ROSPA, Cannon House, The Priory, Queensway, Birmingham, B4 6BS (tel: 021-233 2461)*.

To prevent slipping in icy weather, it is possible to get shoe chains which can be worn over ordinary walking shoes. These cost £6.50 a pair (to blind customers) including postage and packing, and are available from the distributors, *Rud Chains Ltd, 1-3 Belmont Road, Whitstable, Kent, CT5 1QJ (tel: Whitstable (0227) 266464)*.

Grooming
In the last few years several beauticians have devoted special attention to the problems of skin care and make-up methods for blind women. Some of the more enterprising local rehabilitation centres invite make-up experts to discuss problems with blind women. But the pioneer in the field has been Eve Gardiner, Directrice of Beauty at Max Factor, who first got interested in the problems of make-up for the blind when she was asked to advise war-blinded women. Over the

years Miss Gardiner has taken an interest in the problems of make-up for visually handicapped people of all ages. She regularly visits some schools to advise teenagers and occasionally goes also to old people's clubs. She has written a guide to basic make-up techniques for the blind, which will be sent free on request – and will also endeavour to answer individual queries by post. Write to her at *Max Factor Ltd, PO Box 3AH, 16 Old Bond Street, London W1A 3AH*.

Hairdressers are sometimes prepared to visit people in their own homes. If enquiries at local shops prove unsuccessful, it might be possible to get the name of a hairdresser prepared to help a blind person unable to get to a salon by writing to *The Guild of Hairdressers, 24 Woodbridge Road, Guildford, Surrey, GU1 1DY*.

Men who prefer not to shave with razors because of their poor sight might like to know that there is quite a wide range of electric shavers sold at a discount through the RNIB.

Taking medicines

There is a medicine dispenser which screws on to a standard medicine bottle and measures out a 5 ml. dose accurately, quickly and without risk of spillage. It can be obtained free from the RNIB.

It is also possible to get medicine labels – with instructions such as 'Take one three times a day' – marked in braille and large print. These are only suitable for fixing on to bottles – they are too big for a small box of pills. These labels are free and should be available from chemists' shops on request. If not, the pharmacist should be able to obtain them for a blind customer from the manufacturer, *Warner Lambert*.

A tablet container designed to help those who have to take medication regularly may also be particularly useful for blind people. The container is slightly larger than the spool of a typewriter ribbon and has twelve separate compartments which will each take one large tablet or two or three small ones. There is a rotating disc cover which gives a distinct click as it is turned to each compartment, and a small knob on the cover to indicate when the last four compartments have been reached. The Doseaid costs £2.25 (discounts given to blind people) and the price includes VAT. It can be obtained from chemists or direct from the manufacturers, *Medaede Products, 81 Holdenhurst Road, Bournemouth, BH8 8EB (tel: Bournemouth (0202) 528732)*.

Eating

A number of people when they first lose their sight find it very difficult to eat without spilling their food, or indeed sometimes find it difficult to locate their food on the plate. One basic technique, which is widely used by sighted friends or relatives, is to treat the plate like a clock face and explain the position of the food accordingly: 'The meat is at 6 o'clock, the potatoes are at 9 o'clock, and there's some peas at 3 o'clock.' For people who retain a little useful vision it is worth remembering that colour contrasts may make it easier for a visually handicapped person to locate food. It is often far easier for a person with very little sight to locate a meal of fish and mashed potatoes when this is served on a brightly coloured plate than on a plain white one. Those who find it difficult not to spill food off their plate may find it helpful to use a plate-guard, a kind of plastic collar that fits round the edge of the plate. These are made by a number of manufacturers, and range in price between £2.50 and £5. The Disabled Living Foundation can give up-to-date details of manufacturers and prices. The DLF or other aid centres can also give information about various cutlery designs which, though made to meet the need of the physically handicapped, might also be easier for some newly blind people to handle.

It is also possible to buy brightly coloured plastic plates which have been specially designed to make it easier for handicapped people to feed themselves without spilling their food. These 'Manoy' plates have a sloping base and a deep rim at one end. They cost about £2 to £3 each, according to size, and can be ordered from *Noran Aids, 71 Humber Road, Beeston, Nottinghamshire (tel: Nottingham (0602) 227008)*. Some of the other goods stocked by Noran Aids are also of use to visually handicapped people – for example the suction egg cup (36p) might be a boon to someone recovering from a cataract operation, who is finding it difficult to judge distances and is therefore likely to knock things over accidentally.

Royal Doulton have produced an attractive – but rather expensive – range of tableware for disabled people in designs that match their own heavy-duty tableware. There are three different sizes of plate, and a good-sized mug with two handles. Prices vary according to design: a large dinner plate costs between £3.10 and £4.60 and the mug costs between £1.60 and £2.44. Lists of local stockists from *Royal Doulton Hotelware, PO Box 302, Orme Street, Burslem, Stoke on Trent ST6 3RB (tel: Stoke-on-Trent (0782) 89131)*.

It can also be helpful to ensure that plates or other utensils do not slip. Non-slip plastic mats in various sizes are made by *Dycem Limited* and obtainable from *Homecraft Supplies, 27 Trinity Road, London SW17 7SF (tel: 01-672 7070).*

Dycem also produces trays with non-slip surfaces and with arched handles, which are easily carried in one hand, so that a blind person still has one hand free for guidance or protection. Plates can also be secured to trays or table-tops with double suction cups which cost £2.10 a dozen and are obtainable from *Grundy's Ltd, 167 Burton Road, Withington, Manchester M20 8LN*.

Keeping warm

Gas heaters are an especially safe and effective form of heating, and some of the models at present on the market are particularly suitable for the visually handicapped. Automatic ignition is very desirable, and spark ignition, although expensive, is the most reliable device when sight is poor. Clear controls located at the top of the fire are also helpful and several models have push button controls. A flame-failure device which stops the gas supply coming on or staying on if the fire is left unlit is a very useful safety measure. Some gas fires have the radiants sealed behind a transparent glass screen. The Valor Unigas radiant/convector fire has all these features and can be fitted in any room that has a suitable outside wall. Because it has a balanced flue it does not need to be fitted into a fireplace with a chimney.

A list of gas fires whose controls can be adapted for easier and safer handling by people with poor sight and/or weak grip in their hands can be obtained on request from any gas showroom. Blind people who find it difficult to light gas appliances may like to get one of the new spark-ignition lighters which need very little pressure and emit clearly audible clicks when lit. These are obtainable from gas showrooms in various models, ranging in price from £4 to £11.

When buying a new electric fire for a visually handicapped person, it is best to choose one without a radiant element, e.g. convector fires. Models with low surface temperatures are advisable so that accidental contact is not likely to be painful! Fan heaters warm a room quickly and give an audible clue to their location. Wall mounted heaters are worth considering as they avoid the danger of trailing flexes – it is possible to obtain oil filled panel-heaters which fix to the wall. If radiant bar fires are used, they should be placed against a wall with as short a flex as possible. The model chosen should have clear controls fitted at the top of the fire. Old models should always be used in conjunction with a fire guard.

Central heating is, of course, the form of heating which poses fewest problems. The only area of difficulty is likely to be in setting the programmer, but a number of these can be adapted with tactile markings (which do not require a knowledge of braille) through the Royal National Institute for the Blind. When installing central heating, the RNIB will advise on the most suitable type of programmer to choose for adaptation.

For more advice on ways of keeping warm see Chapter 18, *Help for the very elderly*.

Housework

Cleaning

There is no reason why blind people should not be able to do their own housework. Sweeping and dusting need to be done very methodically; the person with sensitive fingers will be able to sense where the dust is. Experienced blind housewives learn to work systematically so that they do not go over the same place twice with a vacuum cleaner or carpet sweeper. When washing floors, the lines of the floor covering – such as tiles – can be used as guides. If the surface is completely smooth, a piece of paper can serve as a guide. It is more effective to work in increasing circles, than to make wide sweeping gestures when cleaning floors or dusting.

Laundry

Most competent blind people manage to wash their clothes, and housewives even do their entire family wash quite satisfactorily by rubbing every item carefully, particularly on areas likely to be especially dirty – such as shirt collars and cuffs. For drying, it is much safer to have a clothes-line which runs along the length of the garden, perhaps starting at one side of the house, than one which extends across the width and is difficult for a blind person to find without bumping into it. A rotary clothes-line has the advantage that the user can stand still and rotate the line in order to hang up the washing. An apron with deep pockets to hold clothes pegs is also useful. There is even a rain warning device, an electronic gadget devised by the technical staff of the RNIB; this is sensitive to moisture so that it will sound a little alarm as a warning to bring in clothes (or the baby) from outside when the first drop of rain falls. This device is available from the RNIB (catalogue no. 9291), price £5.81, or with an extension lead (catalogue no. 9345), price £6.28.

Washing machines: An automatic machine is obviously easier for a blind housewife than a twin-tub, and braille discs to replace the ordinary dials can usually be obtained from the manufacturer. If they can not supply them, then the technical department of the RNIB may be able to help. The RNIB also has a very helpful leaflet giving details of manufacturers of domestic electrical equipment. This leaflet shows how they can be contacted to find out details of modifications to their equipment.

In 1981 Candy brought out a washing machine which was stated to have been designed for the blind in co-operation with technicians from the Italian Institute for the Blind. The machine has all controls marked with large embossed letters. It costs £169.00 including VAT and delivery. For more details contact *Hamilton Electrical Distributors, Hamilton House, Chesford Grange, Woolston, Warrington, Cheshire WA1 4RQ (tel. Pudgate (0925) 821700).*

Irons: Two kinds of adaptations are available. Braille dials can be fitted to all modern irons; when buying an iron the retailer should be asked to contact the manufacturers to see if there is a stock of braille discs available. Many manufacturers have a small stock of them, if they are not available from the factory, the retailer should be asked to remove the ordinary dial and send it to the RNIB's technical department so that a braille equivalent can be provided. In addition to the braille discs, some blind people might be grateful for an additional safety device provided by Hoover, on request, to their steam irons. Hoover will fit, free of charge, a heat muff made of special heat resistant material round the outer edge of the sole plate, so that a blind user cannot inadvertently touch the hot base. The June 1981 edition of *Which?* carried some useful guidelines on choosing an iron for a visually handicapped person.

Sewing
Self-threading needles, where the thread is pushed through a spring in the top of the 'eye', can be bought at most good haberdashery stores, but they are also available free from the RNIB. Some people prefer to

use a needle-threader with ordinary needles as they find the self-threading needles can sometimes break the cotton. Needle-threaders should be easily obtainable at good haberdashers, and are also available free from the RNIB. One device which a number of *In Touch* listeners have recommended is the 'Handi-thread', a plastic gadget which not only threads the needle but also gets the needle eye in the right position. The 'Handi-thread' costs 60p (plus 15p postage) from the maker, *Thomas Mayers, 1 Highview Avenue North, Brighton BN1 8WR*.

Some people with poor sight may find it helpful to use the 'invisible' thread made from monofilament nylon and claimed by the manufacturer to match most colours of material. Peri-Lusta Supersoft invisible thread is available in two tones, natural for light fabrics and smoke for dark colours. It should be available from most large haberdashers, or from the makers, *Peri-Lusta Ltd, Leek, Staffs, ST13 8HE*. Most good haberdashers will also stock Wunderweb, a material adhesive which can be used to fasten zips, waistbands or hems into position without any fine sewing. Tape measures, marked with metal eyelets, are available from the RNIB.

A garment shortener to help a blind or partially-sighted person to turn up a hem accurately had been designed by the late Henry Shear who was for many years the Aids and Gadgets Officer of the Jewish Blind Society. It can be made easily by the average handyman in semi-rigid sheet plastic or aluminium, and will measure hems up to four inches deep. Instructions for making and using the device can be obtained from the *Jewish Blind Society's Day Centre, Robert Zimbler House, 91-3 Stamford Hill, London N16 5TP (tel. 01-800 5672)*.

Many blind people manage to use sewing machines without any adaptations. Electric sewing machines, which leave both hands free are obviously the best choice; and at least one manufacturer has produced a machine specially adapted for the physically handicapped, which also might be useful for some visually handicapped people. The machine is the Bernina 830H, and is available from the *Bogod Machine Company, 50-2 Great Sutton Street, London EC1Y 0DJ*.

Other manufacturers do not have specially adapted machines, but Husqvarna has a blind kit which can be added to the Viking 6270 machine; this comprises an edge guide, slit eye self-threading needles, brailled knobs and a cassette of instructions. Husqvarna have also produced a self-threading sewing machine needle, which should fit most standard sewing machines which take a needle with a shaft that has one flat edge. For further details contact Alan Summers at *Husqvarna's Service Department, Unit 22, Britannia Estate, Leagrave Road, Luton (tel. Luton (0582) 422333)*.

Mrs Ve Appleby has had quite a lot of experience teaching dressmaking to blind students, and has evolved a number of helpful techniques which she would be happy to pass on to any other teachers or students who write to her (enclosing stamped, addressed envelope) at *3 Shepherds Mead, Burgess Hill, Sussex, RH15 8AS*.

Knitting

A limited number of large-print knitting patterns are produced by Wendy Wools. They are available from local Wendy Knit Shops or direct from *Department CP, Carter and Parker Ltd, Guiseley, Yorkshire, LS20 9PD* (send a 10p postal order).

Individual knitting patterns could be enlarged by the Partially Sighted Society's photographic enlargement service, but this costs about 90p a sheet. Details from the Society's business manager, *Eric Howells, 40 Wordsworth Street, Hove*.

It is possible to get knitting patterns recorded on to tape by one of the tape reading services (see page 171) or brailled by one of the transcription services (see page 145).

There is a cassette entitled 'Better knitting made easier' by Audrie Stratford, an experienced knitter who has recorded her own book of instructions for knitting methods and designs that should be easy even for an inexperienced blind person to follow. The cassette can be borrowed free of charge from the *Jewish Blind Society's Day Centre*.

A print version of the book can be obtained (price £2) from *Audrie Stratford, The Bennals, 13 Chase Avenue, Kings Lynn, Norfolk*.

Keeping in touch

Telling the time

A striking clock has the advantage of being a mobility aid (see page 125) as well as a timekeeper. Striking clocks are rarely portable, however, so the RNIB stock a range of clocks and watches suitable for people with poor sight. The clocks, which range in price from £3.55 to £23.70, do not have a glass cover on their faces, but have specially strengthened hands, whilst the hours are indicated by raised dots and the quarters by double dots. An electric alarm clock is also obtainable. Eleven styles of watches are available, ranging in price from £16.68 to

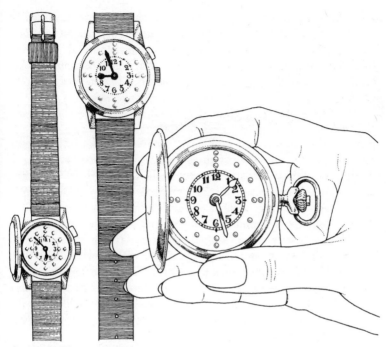

Small and large wristwatch with tactile markings, and hinged glass cover. The markings on the pocket watch may be easier for newly blind people to feel.

£32.63. All look exactly like an ordinary wristwatch, but the glass front is hinged and opens up when a push button is pressed. The strengthened hands can then be felt. It is worth noting that it is easier to open the watch when this push button is at the 2 o'clock position rather than – as on some models – at 6 o'clock. Watches require a more sensitive touch than clocks if they are to be used effectively. The easiest type to use is the pocket watch (£17) followed by the larger wristwatches. Full details are available from the RNIB, who will be glad to advise on a suitable choice. In some areas the local voluntary society for the blind may keep a selection of clocks and watches for local people to examine.

In the last year, however, an increasingly popular choice for many blind people needing a timepiece, has been the 'talking clock', a Japanese-made alarm clock which will 'speak' the time whenever a small knob is pressed. The clock also has a digital display, and it is not much bigger than a cigarette packet. It is available generally in shops for about £40, but quite a number of voluntary societies for the blind have bought them in bulk and are selling them at concession prices to local blind people. Details of stockists from *Sharp Electronics (UK) Ltd, Sharp House, Thorp Road, Manchester M10 9BE (tel. 061-205 2333)*.

Telephoning

Blind people can solve the problem of dialling in various ways. Some have the dial notched at the figures 4 and 7, which makes it easier to find not only these but also the rest of the digits; others, including professional telephonists, manage to cope quickly and efficiently without any markings using a system described in a leaflet called 'Instructions for Telephone Dialling', and available free from the RNIB. People with some residual vision may find it easier to use a wall-mounted telephone, so that the dial is at eye level. Those who find it difficult to see the numerals on the dial may find it helps to stick on an enlarged numeral dial ring. This has large clear black numbers on a white background, and the ring, which is self-adhesive, fits around the dial of an ordinary telephone. It is available (price 40p) from the local telephone sales office.

Another large-print telephone dial, printed with large white numbers on a black background – it is really a self-adhesive label designed to fit neatly around a telephone dial – costs 8p each, (but send a stamped, self-addressed envelope when ordering) from *Surrey Voluntary Association for the Blind, Rentwood, School Lane, Fetcham, Surrey KT22 9JX (tel. Leatherhead (03723) 77701)*.

Dialling is easier with the push-button telephone. These cost £2 extra per quarterly rental; but some blind people, who get confused with the ordinary dial, find it easier to cope when the numbers are arranged in rows of three and only need to be pressed. An additional facility for those who have shaky hands as well as failing eyesight is the press-button finger guide which effectively separates the numeral keys so that it is impossible to touch two at once. This costs 80p and is available from the local telephone sales office.

Additional facilities available with push-button telephones are the callmakers which can automatically dial numbers that have been previously selected and stored by the user. The callmakers range from the Mono callmaker which can be pre-set to call one number at the press of a button to the Tape callmaker which can store up to 400 numbers. Possibly the most useful callmaker for the average domestic user is the X-press callmaker which can store up to ten numbers. Then all that is necessary when wanting to call the doctor, neighbour or whoever is to recall that the doctor is on no. 1 key, the neighbour on no. 2, and so on – and press! The additional quarterly rental for the X-press callmaker is £6.

A blind person who wants to make notes in braille while using the telephone needs to have both hands free. There is available a telerest, a gadget which supports the telephone receiver on the shoulder. This costs £1.64 from office equipment stores or can be obtained direct from *Stricklands & Co. (Blackfriars) Ltd, 3-11 The Cut, London SE1 8LA*.

A better, though more expensive, solution is to get from British Telecom an auralite headset: this is a lightweight earpiece that plugs into a socket on the telephone, and leaves both hands free. The telephone needs to be adapted and, as well as the £10 installation charge, there is also an additional quarterly rental of £8. Many blind people also like to be able to record messages straight on to a tape recorder. Local telephone sales offices keep lists of recording equipment suitable for connection to the telephone and this should be available on request. British Telecom is concerned that any recording equipment is compatible with the user's particular telephone installation, and any equipment used to record telephone conversations needs to have a connector suitable for the telephone socket. British Telecom does not approve of devices using rubber sucker induction coils. Anyone buying equipment with which they plan to record from the telephone is advised to explain to the manufacturer or supplier so that they can ensure the recorder is approved by British Telecom, and has the special connector fitted. British Telecom will charge for installing the equipment, and also ask for a small additional rental for maintaining the connection in good order. The time taken for installation varies from one area to another, but local telephone managers would look sympathetically at an application from a blind subscriber to have this equipment installed. A Revox telephone adaptor for recording calls is available (price £5.17) from the Foundation for Audio Research and Services for Blind People.

The STD book is available in braille from the RNIB in two volumes (catalogue no.28551/2) and a large print version is available from the Partially Sighted Society (price £1.50). For those who read Moon, the Moon Society will make up personal lists of telephone numbers.

Other ways of making notes of telephone numbers for non-braille writers are noted on page 160.

Post
Blind people pay no postal charges on braille material, but are not exempted from paying postage on typed letters or personal tapes or cassettes. However, tapes and cassettes such as those made by talking newspapers or tape services for the blind are eligible for free postage. Anything to be sent free must carry the special label marked 'Articles for the Blind' which is supplied free by the RNIB. This enables braille letters, books and papers to be posted free of charge within the British Isles and by surface mail abroad. Apparatus, such as white sticks, braille clocks, and guide dog harnesses can be sent post free by recognised organisations dealing with the blind. More details of postal concessions are given on a free leaflet supplied by the RNIB.

Shopping
The ideal shop for a visually handicapped person is the old-fashioned corner shop where the proprietor knows his customers and their needs well. But such shops are diminishing in number; and blind people on a limited income may be reluctant to pay the higher prices they charge in comparison with the supermarkets.

Supermarkets and self-service shopping present obvious difficulties to a person unable to see the goods displayed. Most of the larger supermarkets and chain-stores expressed themselves, in response to an inquiry from the *In Touch* office, as willing to help blind customers, if they would make their needs known to an assistant or supervisor. Several stores would ask an assistant to help the customer with their purchases; and a number, including Sainsbury's, Marks & Spencer and Littlewoods, allow guide-dogs to accompany their owners around the shop, despite their general ban on dogs in food departments. It obviously is advisable, if at all possible, for blind shoppers to avoid busy periods when assistants are under great pressure. It is also useful to remember that most supermarkets have a wide selection of goods sold under their own brand name. These are invariably cheaper than the branded goods of other companies and often the contents are identical in quality and quantity. Consistent buying of such goods is the most economical way of shopping and can compensate blind shoppers for being unaware of special offers.

Guide dog owners who sometimes may be refused admission to food shops because of hygiene regulations, should be aware that late in 1976 the Minister for the Disabled, Alfred Morris, announced that food shops and restaurants which normally prohibit dogs should be encouraged to make an exception in the case of guide dogs, and a circular to this effect was sent by the Department of Health to all local authorities. This recommended that notices prohibiting dogs from food premises should specifically exempt guide-dogs. Stick-on notices – suitable for display in shop windows – are obtainable free from the Guide Dogs for the Blind Association.

Money matters

Banks
In recent years the banks have shown quite a lot of interest in ways of helping their visually handicapped customers. All the banks will issue their customers with templates to fit over their cheque books to enable them to fill out the required details in the correct places. In addition all the main high street banks will undertake to send statements in braille – and Lloyds will also provide large print statements on request. Barclays, Trustee Savings Banks and National Westminster will undertake correspondence in braille with a blind customer – National Westminster have in fact trained some of their staff in braille for this purpose.

Ways of calculating
An abacus might help blind people who take the trouble to master it. Those who use it say it is unequalled for the straightforward mathematical processes of addition, subtraction, multiplication and division. The model supplied by the RNIB is roughly the size of a pocket wallet. It costs 85p and full instructions on how to use it are available in both inkprint and braille. The Tape Recording Service for the Blind has instructions and exercises in the use of the abacus available for loan on two C90 cassettes. It is also possible to get calculators with audible outputs, though their prices make them uneconomical for the blind housewife to check her bill in the super-markets! Details of these calculators can be obtained from *Telesensory Systems Inc, PO Box 286, London W4 4EN* which has produced the Speech Plus Talking Calculator – price £255; or a talking calculator

for £85 (plus VAT) is available from *Panasonic Business Equipment, 107-109 Whitby Road, Slough, Berkshire.*

Insurance
Many visually handicapped people have found it difficult to get insurance companies to accept them for householders', travel or other policies at normal rates. The RNIB, with the co-operation of the Bremar Insurance Services Ltd, has got a number of leading insurance companies to agree in principle that a person whose only disability is a visual handicap should be able to take out insurance policies of all kinds at normal rates. Visually handicapped people who wish to get insurance cover should first contact the Finance Secretary of the RNIB.

Looking after babies
Quite a number of visually handicapped women, including totally blind ones, have successfully brought up their own families. There is no national organisation at the moment which links up blind mothers in an attempt to exchange ideas and experiences, although individual blind mothers have been quick to say that it is usually another blind mother who has given them the most useful advice. A set of notes on practical points such as coping with feeding, nappy-changing and the general care of babies and toddlers has been prepared by a totally blind mother with two children, and is available on request from the RNIB.

In addition a telephone advisory service for blind mothers (and also for the parents of blind children) has been set up by Gillian Hinds, who is a blind mother with two children and the wife of one of the RNIB's education advisors. Mrs Hinds is happy to be contacted at any time either by parents or health visitors or others concerned with the care of blind parents or their children. Her telephone number is Northampton (0604) 407726.

One problem which blind parents with young babies have to cope with is a way of transporting the child safely. Many opt for the various kinds of baby slings that have now become popular, as this leaves their hands free for coping with their own mobility aid – be it a long cane or a guide dog. But it is also possible now to get an adapted pram specially designed for blind parents which can be pulled along with the aid of a harness strapped to a parent's body. This adaptation to a pram is the brain-child of Keith Goldson, a blind man with a blind wife and three children, who had experienced the difficulties of coping simultaneously with small children and pushchairs. The adaptation to the pram (reconditioned Silver Cross models are being used) is being carried out by a sheltered workshop in Slough. Details from *Bob Underwood* at *Speedwell Enterprises, Northampton Avenue, Slough SL1 3BP (tel: Slough (0753) 72249)*.

The first blind mother to use one of these prams is Mrs Gail Guest of Ashford, Middlesex, who is happy to give details of the pram to anyone who is interested (tel: Ashford (07842) 41991).

There is a limited amount of literature for new parents in braille. The Scottish Braille Press produce all the BMA's pamphlets such as 'You and Your Pregnancy', 'Common Ailments in Babies', 'Common Ailments in Toddlers' and Gateshead Public Libraries have produced a tape version of 'The Baby Book' which can be borrowed through the public library system by anyone living elsewhere in Britain. The La Leche League, which is an American organisation set up to encourage mothers with breast feeding, has some material on tape or in braille. Contact *Mrs Tarin Brokenshire, PO Box BM 3424, London WC1V 6XX* or telephone 01-404 5011 for details of nearest group.

Another helpful cassette, 'Being a Blind Mother' (part of a series made for the Medical Recording Service by Jill Allen) can be obtained direct from her at *59 Silversea Drive, Westcliff-on-Sea, SSO 9XB (tel: Southend (0702) 74059)*.

Mrs Allen, who lost her sight a year before the birth of her daughter, feels it would be mutually beneficial if blind mothers could form an association in order to exchange useful information, as she has found that doctors and health visitors so rarely have to cope with a blind mother that they are not able to be very helpful about the practical problems she meets.

★ *To help a blind mother keep track of an active baby or toddler, tie small bells to child's ankle.*
(Julie Welsh)

7 In the kitchen

There is very little equipment specially designed for a blind house-wife, but many of the basic ideas of good kitchen design and planning are not only equally valid for a blind housewife, but can sometimes constitute necessities rather than luxuries. A useful service offering information about equipment for disabled housewives is provided by the Disabled Living Foundation, which has a permanent exhibition centre at 346 Kensington High Street, London W14 8NS. The exhibition can be visited by appointment only. In addition the Foundation has an information service to deal with queries of all kinds concerning aids and equipment for disabled users. The foundation will answer queries sent by letter, but asks that as much information as possible is given about the exact needs of the disabled person. For a list of similar centres in other cities see *Useful Addresses* on page 271.

General points to bear in mind when planning or adapting a kitchen for someone with little or no sight is that a worktop alongside the cooker – ideally at the same height – will make it easier and safer to transfer pans; plenty of cupboards and storage space will enable equipment and food to be stored neatly and methodically. It is safer for cupboards to have sliding doors rather than doors which can inadvertently be left open and prove a hazard for a blind person. A pull-out board with holes to take mixing bowls is also very useful. It is probably best for a visually handicapped person to have a kitchen floor covering which is light in colour and plain in design. This makes it easier for someone with limited vision to see something which has dropped on the floor; it also helps to use kitchen equipment in easily distinguished colours – contrasting rather than matching the working surfaces.

Good lighting in the kitchen is essential if a person with any residual vision is to make good use of it when cooking or preparing food. Striplights or spot lights that illuminate the working area can be very helpful (see page 116 for more details).

Organisation

Storage
More than anyone else, a visually-handicapped person has to learn to

be methodical and tidy in every aspect of work in a kitchen. It is no luxury to have as many cupboards as possible, placed sensibly in relation to the work to be done with the material stored, because this makes it easier to remember where things are and cuts down the amount of walking back and forth carrying materials. Cupboards at eye-level can be dangerous if they have doors that open outwards; it would be much better to have sliding doors fitted. If storage space within the cupboards is so organised that different types of things are always kept separately, this will be of great help. If, for example, tinned vegetables are always kept on one shelf and fruit on another this prevents one possible confusion. Equally, if the blind shopper gets into the habit of buying baked beans in large sizes and curried beans by the same manufacturer in a medium or small size, this also helps to distinguish the contents. Many blind housewives use different-shaped containers for staple products such as flour, sugar, and so on. Hanging baskets which fit under shelves can be very useful to give extra storage space and help to separate items. Dividers in drawers help to keep small items clearly separated. Carousel shelves which can be fitted into cupboards to swing out when the doors are opened save a lot of bending and searching.

The more a kitchen is planned to prevent unnecessary movements, the easier it will be; for example, if the rubbish bin is next to the sink, plates can be scraped right over it and then put into the washing-up bowl. If the tin-opener is kept in a drawer – or wall-mounted – near the cupboard where the tins are stored, this will save time and energy. Knives can be stored safely on the wall behind the worktop by using a wall mounted magnetic holder.

Labelling
Housewives who know braille can get magnetic rubber strips from the RNIB which can be marked in braille and used over and over again to distinguish the contents of tins. Self-adhesive plastic labelling foil, which can be embossed in braille by machine or hand frame and then cut to size, is an excellent material for labelling. It is available from the RNIB in black, which produces a white dot, or clear for use on instruments or for fixing over lettering when it is important not to obliterate the printing underneath. Small self-adhesive labels for brailling are available free from the RNIB, as are domestic labels with eyelet holes, suitable for use in a deep freeze.

For non-braillists it is possible to get labels embossed in Moon from the RNIB's Moon branch. But people who cannot read either embossed script often work out their own labelling methods, using tactile markers ranging from rubber bands to magnetic letters available from toy shops. An invaluable source of ideas about methods of labelling is Jessica Finch who has devised her own exhibition of labelling methods for the visually handicapped. Further details from Mrs Finch at *24 Norwich Street, Cambridge* (see also page 160).

Large appliances

Cookers
Totally blind people, as well as those with varying degrees of visual handicap, have worked equally well with gas and electric cookers. Most housewives who lose their sight are happiest to continue using their familiar cooker. The only modification that most people need is to have some kind of tactile marker for the controls. It is possible to get braille dials to mark the oven regulo for almost all cookers – and even non-expert braillists can often learn to read these. The braille discs can be fitted by arrangement with either the gas or electricity showroom.

The RNIB's technical department has produced an information sheet detailing which gas and electric cookers can be easily fitted with braille controls. This leaflet also points out that while it is not practicable to adapt most cooker oven timers for use by blind people, there is one type of oven timer which is suitable for blind people with good hearing and a sensitive touch to use without any adaptation. A separate information sheet (also obtainable from the RNIB's technical department) gives details of this automatic oven timer and a list of gas and electric cookers which incorporate this device.

In addition to braille, people have used a variety of raised marking devices, from those such as split shot and araldite which is difficult to fix, to the relatively new American substance Hi-marks, which is bright orange and easily seen by people with a little sight (see page 160 for details).

It is impossible, given the variety of cooker models available, to make specific recommendations about gas or electric cookers that are particularly easy for blind people to use. The gas and electricity boards both employ advisers for the disabled whose help can be sought. When choosing a cooker for a blind person it is useful to look out for features such as clear controls at the front of the hob, ideally with all 'off' positions in the same direction. It is very helpful for a partially sighted cook to have a light in the oven and it is no luxury for a visually handicapped person to pay the little extra needed to get an oven that has a self-cleaning lining! Drop-down oven doors and non-tip shelves are also a boon.

Some electric oven controls give an audible click when turned to the 'off' position, and some gas cookers have 'click' settings, particularly for simmering. A number of modern gas cookers are now lit by spark ignition and for other models it is possible to get spark-ignition gas lighters which need very little pressure and emit clearly audible clicks when lit. Some gas cookers which are lit by spark ignition also have a re-ignition device built into the system which automatically relights a burner if it is accidentally extinguished. A number of cookers have this re-ignition device only in the oven, but it is possible to find models which have it on the hob as well.

Microwave ovens have certain advantages for blind cooks. They remain cool in use as do the utensils in which food is cooked, so there is no risk of accidental burns when handling food in and out of the oven. The microwave ovens are small and can be placed on a work top so that they are at eye-level, and the cook does not need to stoop. The controls are usually simple to operate and on some models operate audibly. But not all microwave ovens have controls that are suitable for brailling, some panels are too complex.

The Toshiba model ER 649 can be brailled to order and Toshiba offers a 15 per cent discount to registered blind or partially sighted customers who buy direct from them at *Toshiba House, Frimley Road, Camberley, Surrey (tel. Camberley (0276) 62222)*. General details about microwave cookers can be obtained from the *Microwave Oven Association, 16a The Broadway, London SW19 1RF (tel. 01-946 3389)*.

Another increasingly popular form of cooking that might appeal to a blind person is the 'slo-cooker' which in various models have come on the market in recent years. These use relatively little fuel and are particularly good for 'all in one meals' like pot-roasts and casseroles which may be easier for a blind cook to prepare and serve than a meal consisting of several different items cooked separately. In addition, a BEAB – approved slo-cooker should never get so hot on the outside as to burn anyone who inadvertently touches it. Available in a price range of approximately £15 to over £30, depending on size, from

Electricity Board showrooms, household goods stores, department stores. Details of manufacturers of slow cookers from the *Electricity Council, 30 Millbank, London SW1P 4RD (tel. 01-834 2333).*

Refrigerators
As with cookers, there is no particular model that is specially suited to the needs of a blind person. If possible it is helpful to have automatic defrosting; but if it is to be defrosted manually it is important to have a deep drip tray. Door storage racks are particularly useful, as is an interior light. Plastic boxes with coloured lids, and brightly coloured plastic bags in plain colours, or in stripes, are obtainable from *Lakeland Plastics, 33 Alexandra Road, Windermere, Cumbria LA23 2BZ.* Although designed for use in freezers they would also be helpful to someone with limited vision trying to distinguish the contents of a refrigerator.

A combined fridge/freezer has great advantages for a blind person. The long-term storage capacity of the freezer not only means that it is possible to cut down on the number of shopping expeditions, which even the most mobile and active blind person can find tiring; but for those less able to look after themselves it gives them the opportunity to store cooked food prepared for them by friends or relatives.

Useful kitchen equipment
The articles listed below are obtainable, unless otherwise specified, from ordinary household hardware shops. Most of the items are basic kitchen equipment, but have features that are particularly useful to cooks with little or no sight.

Bread-cutting box: This has been designed by the RNIB and is available in right- and left-handed models at a price of £2.17 (catalogue no. 9442 and 9442L). There is an adjustable slide to help determine the thickness of the slice.

Bread-cutting aid: A smaller slicing aid can be made from a stiff strip of aluminium measuring about 2in. by 15in. This can be bent into a horseshoe shape with three sharp prongs on the inner surface of each side formed by making an indentation on the outside. This can be placed over a loaf of bread to act as a guide for the breadknife, and the prongs grip the side of the loaf to prevent it from slipping as the slices of bread are cut. This aid is not available commercially; it was devised by Henry Shear who, until his death in 1981, was Aids and Gadgets Officer of the Jewish Blind Society. Instructions for making the guide can be obtained from the *JBS Day Centre*.

Butter gauge: For those who like to measure their fat by cutting the standard pack into four equal portions, the Jewish Blind Society provides the pattern for a butter gauge (which it claims can be easily made) to measure 50, 100, 150 and 200 grammes. This too was devised by Henry Shear. Instructions for making this aid can be obtained from the *JBS Day Centre*.

Chopper: A collapsible Swiss-made bell-shaped vegetable chopper keeps fingers away from the sharp zig-zag blades; these are operated by a plunger. The dome folds back for easy cleaning, and there is a detachable chopping base. It costs £4.95 at household goods stores; details of local stockists from the distributor: *Zyliss (UK) Ltd, Rodney House, Castlegate, Nottingham (tel. 0602 582161)*.

Chopping board: It may be easier for people with limited vision to see what they are cutting if the colour of the chopping board contrasts sharply with the food on it. White polyethylene chopping boards are available from catering equipment shops, and have the additional advantage of being easier to clean than conventional wooden boards. They are available in two sizes: 12in. by 9in. by ½in. (£2.80 plus VAT) and 18in. by 12in. by ½in. (£4.95 plus VAT). Details of stockists from *S.J.H. Row & Sons Ltd, 5 Stepfield, Industrial Area East, Witham, Essex (tel. Witham (0376) 511101)*.

Chip basket: Useful for cooking large vegetables – when cooked, they can simply be lifted out of the saucepan without the need to drain away boiling water – as well as for deep frying. Available from household goods stores; costs £1.55 at John Lewis branches.

Colander: Easiest to use for draining vegetables, spaghetti and so on is a long-handled colander, which will cost £2.50 to £4 from household goods stores or catering equipment shops.

Cooker: The Rima 3 in 1 is an electric pan, slow cooker and deep fryer combined, with a capacity of 1.5 litres (just over 2½ pints). It costs approximately £20 and is available from Electricity Board showrooms and branches of John Lewis, Currys, Argos, Comet and Tesco and mail order companies.

Dispenser: A medicine dispenser which attaches direct to the bottle (catalogue no. 9284), is available free from the RNIB.

Dispenser: For drinks, see *Vacuum flasks*, page 93.

Dispensers (for dry goods): Kitchen dispensers suitable for tea, instant coffee, granulated sugar or washing powder (and other dry goods wanted in spoonfuls) are available. Those made by Arthur Douglas come in two sizes and in bright colours, and are easily dismantled for cleaning. They cost £1.80 for the ¼lb capacity, and £2.30–£2.50 for the ½lb size. Details of local stockists from *Arthur Douglas, Nields Factory, Penarth Road, Cardiff CF1 7TT (tel. (0222) 387145)*.

Drinkups: These are Pyrex glasses in brightly coloured plastic holders, which are easier to see than ordinary glassware – as well as being suitable for hot liquids. They cost around £1–£1.25 in household goods shops.

Egg boiling ring: A simple circular rack, with a central handle, into which up to half a dozen eggs can be placed. This is very simple to lower and raise from the saucepan. Made by Skyline, and available from household goods shops, it costs around £1.64.

Egg poaching ring: When frying or poaching an egg, it is helpful to place it within a ring – usually made of aluminium – so that the rim of the ring acts as a guide for the spatula when it is time to take out the egg. The ordinary commercial rings have no handles, but the RNIB have produced their own model (catalogue no. 9070); on one side of the ring there is a useful little handle, angled to guide the hand to the exact centre of the ring. This cost 25p.

Egg separator: A simple plastic gadget which can, like a tea strainer, be placed over a cup or small basin. When an egg is cracked over it, the base of the separator keeps the yolk, while the white seeps through the slits in the sides. Made by Nutbrown, available at household goods shops, this costs about 76p.

Eye dropper bottles: Small quantities of liquid (e.g. flavouring essences) can be dispensed through eye dropper bottles which have not previously been used for medicines. These are obtainable from chemists for approximately 30p.

Food preparation system: The Braun Multiquick has a basic chopper unit (ZK1) for about £23; there is also a blender/liquidiser attachment (ZK3). If this is sold separately it costs around £11, or the two together (ZK2) cost approximately £27. There is another attachment, a slicer/shredder (ZK4) which costs around £14, or the Multiquick Tri-Set (ZK5), which is the complete set, costs in the region of £40. The controls are easy to operate by someone without sight and the equipment is particularly safe for blind people to use as it will not function at all unless it is completely locked. Available at retailers of electrical goods; details of local stockists from *Braun Electric (UK) Ltd, Dolphin Estate, Windmill Road, Sunbury-on-Thames, Middlesex (tel. Sunbury 85611)*.

Funnels: Ordinary kitchen funnels are very helpful to a blind cook who wants to pour without risk of spillage. It is worth buying a number of different sizes – the largest will take rice, lentils and other small solid foods as well as liquids.

For filling a hot water bottle (or for any other task where there is a danger of liquid bubbling over the top) a safety funnel with a collar round the top of its stem, which will allow air to escape, is best. These funnels are available with a 3½in. diameter (21p) and 6¼in. diameter (around 40p) from household goods stores such as Boots, Timothy Whites, Sainsbury. Details of local stockists from Arthur Douglas Ltd (for address and phone number, see *Dispensers (for dry goods)*, page 86).

Gas lighter: A click-ignition model is probably most useful, as it gives an audible signal. Lighters are available from most gas showrooms, in a price range from around £4 to about £11 (the click-ignition type costs in the region of £7.50).

Harbenware dry-pan: This is an unusually designed frying pan; it is quite deep and has a central funnel through whose holes heat circulates when cooking. The pan is lined with non-stick material, needs very little fat and is claimed by the manufacturers to revolutionise the cooking of sausages, bacon, eggs, chips and other foods that usually require a lot of fat. It will cook only a limited quantity at once, and timing and temperature control are very important. But as it will only cook when the lid is on, and uses so little fat, a blind person can fry with no fear of spurting fat. The Dry-Pan is made in various sizes; the smallest costs £9.12 plus VAT and postage and packing. It is only available direct from the manufacturer, *Harbenware Ltd, Hanover Mill, Fitzroy Street, Ashton-under-Lyne, Lancashire OL7 0JF (tel. 061-330 3081)*.

Kettles: Electric kettles with an automatic switch-off are valuable, but some people prefer an audible signal to indicate when the water is boiling. Swan makes two such models, each with a three-pint capacity. The Autosonic, a shiny chrome kettle, buzzes when it comes to the boil; it costs approximately £24. The Swan whistling electric kettle, available in cream, red or brown, has the upper and lower water level limit indicated by bars inside. The element in this cannot be replaced, but each kettle has a two-year guarantee. This costs around £10.50. Both these kettles are available from high street stores such as Rumbelows, Argos, the Co-op and Comet or Macro.

The Redring Autoboil is an electric kettle shaped like a vacuum jug. It is light and easy to handle, and has a plastic surface which never gets hot enough to burn. It has a capacity of three pints, but can safely boil as little as one cupful of water at a time. This costs approximately £20 from department stores, electrical goods shops, Electricity Board showrooms.

Knife rack: A magnetic knife rack is a safe and convenient way of storing sharp knives. Available in various sizes, and costing about £4.95 for a 12in. rack or £6.25 for one 22in. in length (plus VAT), they should be available at catering equipment stores. If not in stock, ask the retailer to order from *M. Gilbert (Greenford) Ltd, 1109 Greenford Road, Greenford, Middlesex (tel. 01-422 6178 or 01-864 3488)*.

Knives: The Swiss Dux carving knife has a detachable guard which can be adjusted to control the width of slices, and can be used for anything from bread to cold meat. For blind customers there is a special price of £9.95 plus 55p postage, direct from *Lesway, 3 Clarendon Terrace, London W9 1BZ (tel. 01-289 7197)*.

A French chef's stainless steel knife is useful for the method of preparing vegetables illustrated on page 97. A Sabatier knife with a riveted handle costs around £6 for the 7in. size from catering equipment stores; some department stores also stock them. Details of local stockists from *Philbar & Co., 56 Wilson Street, London EC2A 2EN (tel. 01-247 4803)*.

Liquid level indicator: An ingenious little device, first developed by a young engineer – Jeffrey Burndrett – to help his blind father. Battery-operated, it consists basically of two sets of prongs made from rhodium plated wire. When the tip of the wire touches something wet, the indicator buzzes. The prongs can easily be hooked over the side of a cup or glass – the shorter wire on the inside if one wants a warning of the vessel filling up to the top, the longer wire inside if one wants to put a little milk or other liquid in the bottom. The wire is untarnishable and can be used in any liquid, hot or cold. The indicator is available from the RNIB (catalogue no. 9485) and costs £2.26.

An adaptation of this indicator – which will vibrate rather than buzz, and so give a tactile signal useful to the deaf-blind – is being developed by the RNIB and should be available soon for about £10.

Measuring jugs: The RNIB sells a Pyrex measuring jug (catalogue no. 9077) with raised markings inside to indicate levels of ¼, ½, ¾ and 1 pint; 97p.

Most department stores, multiples and independent hardware stores sell a polypropylene measuring jug with clear black markings; the 1-litre size costs around £1.25, and there is also a smaller size available. Details of local stockists from *Stewart Plastics Ltd, Purley Way, Croydon CR9 4HS (tel. 01-686 2231)*.

Measuring spoons: There is a particularly useful set available in white plastic, with flat-based spoons that will not tip. There are four spoons in the holder, each measuring imperial at one end and the metric equivalent at the other. Capacity ranges from ¼ teaspoonful to 1 tablespoonful. The set costs around £1.50 from household goods stores; details of local stockists from *Plysu Housewares Ltd, Woburn Sands, Milton Keynes MK17 8SE (tel. Milton Keynes (0908) 582311)*.

Milksaver pan: This is a 1-pint capacity milk saucepan, with a separate anti-boil device which fits into the pan. If used on medium or gentle heat, it should not boil over. It costs approximately £7 from mail order firms such as Marshall Cavendish, but there are special terms for blind customers buying direct from *Brier Housewares, Unit 1, Excelsior Works, Mucklow Hill, Halesowen B62 8EP (tel. 021-501 2807; ask for Mr Scott)*.

Milk-saver: A round disc of ovenproof glass which is placed in the bottom of the pan and rattles when the milk is coming to the boil. On a gentle heat, the milk will then not boil over. The audible signal is a valuable warning, but some people find it a nuisance to have a heavy disc in the pan when trying to pour hot milk into a cup. This Solidex milk-saver is available from household goods stores, John Lewis branches, Boots or through Selfridges Mail Order Department, London W1. It costs around £1.10.

Non-slip material and mats: To stop things slithering about on worktop or table, and thus make food preparation (and consumption) safer and easier. 'Grippistrip' is made in five colours (red, blue, green, yellow and white), and costs £7 for a two-metre length 200mm (8in.) wide (other sizes are available). 'Anchorpads' are available in red, blue and green, and cost from £3.70 for a pad 10in. by 7in. to £4.40 for a pack of four drink coasters, from *Homecraft Supplies, 27 Trinity Road, London SW17 7SF (tel. 01-672 7070/1789)*.

Optics: Those used for dispensing spirits in public houses are another useful aid to pouring. A set of optics costs about £5 at catering equipment stores, though a friendly publican might be able obtain one more cheaply through the trade.

Scales: The best possible scales for a totally blind cook are the old-fashioned balance kind with individual weights that are easily distinguished. Prestige model 951 costs £19.45, and comes with ½oz, 1oz, 2oz, 4oz, ½lb and 1lb weights. On some of the larger weights the markings are raised, and can be 'read' by touch.

Weylux Rex scales cost £20.50 (plus VAT), and the weights – which can be ordered separately – are £7.20 for imperial and £8.80 for metric. Available from Timothy Whites, department stores and mail order firms such as Marshall Cavendish. Details of local stockists from *H. Fereday & Sons, 31-49 Holloway Road, London N7 8JT*.

Viking Scales: the standard domestic model 405m costs £24.50 plus £7.50 for imperial weights, and £9.50 for metric. The manufacturers are *F.J. Thornton & Co., Jenner Street, Wolverhampton WV2 2AE (tel. Wolverhampton (0902) 52390).*

Most domestic kitchen scales use a balance and dial, and a partially sighted cook may find it helpful to use wall-mounted scales at eye level. It is worth shopping around for a model with a clear dial. For cooks who cannot see even the clearest dial, it is possible to get some models – particularly those with an exposed dial and pointer – adapted. This will be done free by the RNIB's technical department.

Waymaster scales are spring balance scales with weights marked in braille and a pointer which can be felt. Available in imperial or metric. Two imperial models are kept in stock: model 424 weighs up to 24oz (1½lb), and is brailled at ¼oz divisions; model 405 weighs up to 5lbs and is brailled at 1oz divisions. The smaller capacity model is probably easier to use as the ¼oz divisions are well spaced on the dial and easier to feel. There are also two metric models, 401K which weighs up to 1 kilo and is brailled at 25g divisions and 425K which weighs up to 2.5 kilos and is brailled at 50g divisions. All Weylux scales cost £6.29 ready adapted, post free, from *Precision Engineering Co. (Reading) Ltd, Meadow Road, Reading RG1 8LB (tel. Reading (0734) 599444).*

Scissors: It is easier, and safer, to cut with a pair of kitchen scissors than with a knife. Some blind people find 'Snips' – all-purpose clippers with blunt ends like secateurs – particularly easy to use. Available from household goods stores for around £2.50.

Slicers: For slicing cucumber or other vegetables (and fruit) thinly, a mandoline-type slicer where the food to be sliced is rubbed over a fixed blade (rather like playing a washboard) is quick and safe. These are also available with an adjustable blade, so that the thickness of the slice can be varied. Available from department stores such as Selfridges and John Lewis, and other retailers of household goods, the adjustable mandoline costs £3.25 plus VAT; a large fixed-blade slicer costs £2.75 plus VAT, and a small one £1.45 plus VAT. Details of local stockists from *Kontinental Housecrafts, Royston Road, Wendens Ambo, Nr Saffron Walden, Essex (tel. Saffron Walden (0799) 40602).*

For slicing boneless meat, bread and other larger items a rotary manual slicer can be useful. A sliding food carrier presses the food to be sliced against the blade which is turned by a handle, so there should be no danger to fingers; and the slices are even in thickness. Various models are available from household goods stores, department stores and Argos, in a price range from around £10 to nearly £20. For details of local stockists of those made by Tower, contact *Service Supply Ltd, Tower House, Harlequin Avenue, Brentford, Middlesex (tel. 01-568 4567)*.

Spatula: A rubber spatula is ideal for clearing all the cake mixture out of a mixing bowl, or custard out of a saucepan.

Splatter guard: This is a circle of wire mesh, closely woven, with a long handle; it fits over almost all makes of frying pan, and prevents hot fat spurting out. It costs about £1 at household goods stores, or from *Selfridges Mail Order Department, London W1*.

Stove mat: A stove mat, made of wire mesh, is a more durable alternative to an asbestos stove mat. It spreads heat evenly under a pan, which makes simmering easier and also ensures the stability of a small saucepan. It costs £1.75, and is available from John Lewis branches, Timothy Whites, Lewis/Selfridge Group, House of Fraser, or direct from *William Levene, 36-8 Willesden Lane, London NW6 7ST (tel. 01-328 1911)*.

Tap turners: Levers to help turn on taps can be a boon to those who find this difficult. The 'Easiturn' for ordinary taps is supplied in pairs – one red, one blue – with braille markings for hot and cold, and cost £2.87 the pair from Homecraft Supplies (for address and telephone see *Non-slip material and mats*, page 68), who also stock tap turners for crystal and supa-taps.

Teapot: For those who worry about inadvertently burning themselves on a hot teapot, a thermal teapot may provide the answer. This is insulated, and does not get hot on the outside (also the tea stays hot longer). It is made in bright colours, and has a wide lid and a short spout so that it is easy to fill and to pour from. Available in two sizes (1pt and 1½pt), it costs around £2.50 or £3 from Woolworths, Boots, Sainsburys, and department stores, or by mail order from *British Mail Corporation, Universal House, Devonshire Street, Ardwick, Manchester M60 6EL (tel. 061-273 8282)*.

Timer: As timing is so crucial for cooks who are not able to see well, a ringer timer is a very valuable piece of equipment. The standard Smiths timer, with raised tactile marks (catalogue no. 9492) was out of stock at the RNIB as this book went to press; but an ordinary kitchen timer can be adapted by using Hi-Marks (see page 160).

Tin opener: Some of the simpler types of tin openers operated by hand from above the tin can be dangerous and difficult to control for people with little or no sight. The same applies to sophisticated electric tin openers. A manually-operated wall-mounted opener is easy to operate, and has the advantage of being fixed in one place and therefore easy to find, but it is likely to be expensive. Prestige make models with magnetic lid lifters; these are available from department stores, household goods shops, Argos etc. and cost from about £5 to around £9.

For those who prefer to open tins on a work- or table-top, Brabantia make a 'butterfly' model which is particularly easy to use by touch alone; there is also a version with a magnetic lid lifter. The standard model costs £2.10, that with the magnet £2.50, at John Lewis branches. Details of local stockists from *Brabantia (UK) Ltd, Blackfriars Road, Nailsea, Bristol BS19 2SB (tel. Bristol (0272) 856661).*

Tongs: There is a variety of kitchen tongs on the market. It is often much easier for a blind person to grip cooking (or cooked) food with a pair of tongs than with a spoon or fork.

Vacuum flasks: There are various designs of vacuum flasks which have pump dispensers instead of the conventional stopper and screwtop lid. This enables someone to pump out hot liquids, a little at a time, without fear of scalding. This kind of flask is ideal for elderly people with unsteady hands who might find it difficult to pour from a heavy flask. Generally available in household goods stores, department stores, Boots, these are made by more than one manufacturer. Thermos make the 'Touch-Top' model in two sizes, and with a choice of metal or plastic casing. The 1-litre size costs £6.55 with a metal cover, £6.95 with plastic cover, from Boots. The 2-litre size costs around £12.75.

Aladdin make the 'Pump-a-Drink' model; this has a capacity of 1 litre, and dispenses about a small cupful each time the top is pressed. It costs around £6.95.

Wall-mounted milk bottle holder: Originally designed by an industrial designer, Alan Pearcey, to help his wife who has spinal trouble, this is also likely to be helpful to blind people – particularly those with eye conditions which make it inadvisable for them to bend down. The Wybend Traditional is a strongly-made steel rack with a durable black nylon coating; it takes four bottles. The number of pints needed is indicated by easily-felt indicator clips, which the milkman can see from a distance. The rack is fixed at a convenient height in holes drilled into the wall. It costs £5.80, plus postage and packing.

There is also a Wybend Special, with an extra rail; it is designed for use by disabled people with clumsy movement. It costs £7.45, plus postage and packing.

The smallest model is a screw-on version, has no indicator clips, and holds only three bottles. It costs £4.14, plus postage and packing.

Further details from *Mr Pearcey, Cut Rose Designs, The Old School, Brandon Bank, Southery, Nr Downham Market, Norfolk PE38 0PU (tel. Brandon Creek (035 376) 271)*.

★ *When using boxes of matches, take a small piece out of the bottom, so its always clear which way up to open it.*
   (Mrs. B. Seekings, Bedford)

★ *As it is sometimes easier for people with limited vision to see things if there is a sharp colour contrast, it might be worthwhile for keen bakers to get their pastry board covered with black formica.*
   (Mrs P.J. Warren, Camberley)

Cookery

For someone who has gone blind, cooking may appear a formidable, if not insuperable, task but many blind women (and men) have learnt to cater not only for themselves, but for their families as well. Probably the best way to learn is at home, on a one-to-one basis with a technical officer, but an excellent alternative is in a group with other blind people and a newly blind person would be well advised to take any rehabilitation course that is available locally.

A newly blind cook needs to learn new methods, rather than new recipes. The suggestions below are based on the regular cookery items broadcast on *In Touch* by Hannah Wright, who worked as a professional cook until she lost her sight. The methods are geared particularly to the needs of a newly blind person and are suggestions for ways of tackling the most common problems rather than a complete guide to cookery for the blind. Suggestions about suitable kitchen equipment are contained in the previous chapter (see page 84), which also gives details of suppliers for equipment mentioned in this chapter.

It is essential for a blind person who is cooking to be able to concentrate on the job without distractions. The sound of the radio or another person's chatter may make it impossible to hear the faint sound that indicates something is coming up to boil. Having all the necessary equipment set out ready on the table or working surface before starting to cook is also recommended. It might also be useful for a visually handicapped cook to wear an apron with deep pockets in which various small tools or gadgets could be kept and easily retrieved when needed.

Preparing food

Weighing and measuring

The American system of using cups for measuring may be easier for blind people to use than adapted spring balance kitchen scales with braille markings. These are specially made by Precision Engineering (for details see page 91) but it needs a good sense of touch as well as a knowledge of braille to read the markings; old-fashioned balance scales with individual weights may be simpler to use. Many blind cooks set aside cups or containers such as yoghurt pots which they know to contain a certain quantity (the standard yoghurt pot holds ¼ pint or 5 fluid ounces) and keep a varied collection of such receptacles for use in weighing. For measuring small quantities of liquid, such as cochineal or other essences, Hannah Wright uses eye dropper bottles from the chemist – ones that have not previously been used for medicaments! A fluted hexagonal teated eye dropper bottle costs about 30p and it can be filled with the help of a funnel or a syringe. A domestic syringe set consisting of a 1 millimetre syringe and a 20 millimetre syringe can be obtained from the RNIB at a concession price of 46p. Instead of guessing the salt or other ingredients usually measured in spoonfuls, Hannah Wright recommends using a set of white plastic flat-bottomed spoons, one end of which measures ¼, ½ and 1 teaspoonful and 1 tablespoonful, and the other has the metric equivalent (see page 89 for details). The medicine dispenser issued free by the RNIB gives an accurate measure of one teaspoonful, but it should never be used for both food and medicines!

Cutting and slicing
Probably the most popular aid to slicing at any *In Touch* cookery demonstration is the Swiss-made 'Dux' slicing knife with a detachable slicing guide that can be adjusted according to the width of slice required. This knife can be used for slicing meat, bread, vegetables and so on (see page 88). Another method which French chefs use to chop vegetables at high speed may be particularly helpful to blind people. This method is adopted by professional cooks to enable them to work at high speed without looking down at their hands. They use a French chef's knife, which has a straight edge tapering to a point, and is between six and twelve inches long. To cut a carrot by this method, it has first to be cut in half lengthways and placed flat side down on the chopping board. The cook's left hand holds the end of the carrot being sliced in such a way that the tips of the fingers are well tucked in, and the second joints of the fingers are vertical. The tip of the knife is placed on the chopping board at the far side of the carrot, resting the side of the blade against the second joints of the fingers. Using the finger joints as a guide the blade is slid down to cut a slice of carrot. For the next slice only the blade, and not the tip of the knife, is raised while the carrot is pushed forward slightly with the thumb of the left hand – and the finger tips are moved back a bit. The tip of the knife remains in position acting as a kind of pivot until the whole carrot is sliced (see illustration on page 97). Although this method seems very

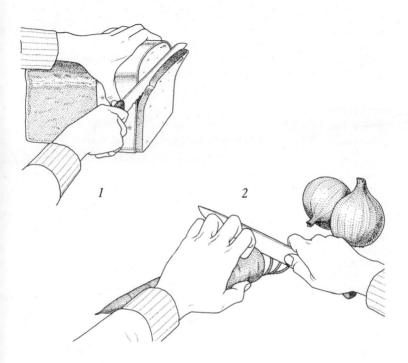

Methods of Slicing
1 *Simple 'do-it-yourself' bread slicing aid, made from a strip of aluminium. (See page 84)*
2 *The French chef's method of slicing*

awkward at first, ease and speed should come with practice. But it is essential to have a proper French chef's knife, which is best bought from a catering equipment shop. A six-inch stainless steel French chef's knife with a riveted handle (glued ones may eventually come apart) would cost about £8.

For those who prefer a chopping device where the fingers do not come into contact with the blade, the Super Autochop – a bell-shaped vegetable chopper – is particularly safe to use. The zig-zag blades, operated by a plunger, are enclosed in a plastic dome, but this can be folded back for easy cleaning. People whose eyes cannot easily tolerate the smell of onions may also like to use this device as the dome completely covers whatever is being chopped and therefore reduces any smell as well as preventing the food from slithering away. Its only disadvantage is that it is impossible to sharpen the blades – so that when they become blunt, the chopper has to be thrown away. (For details see page 85.)

Peeling potatoes
No one has come up with the perfect method for peeling potatoes, but a number of ideas have been put forward by blind cooks.

1. Boil with the skin on. When cooked and drained, hold the potato in a cloth and nip up a little piece of skin between paring knife and thumb and pull it towards you. The skin will come away in large pieces, except where there is an eye to be gouged out. Because of the time taken in peeling, this method is suitable only for small quantities, otherwise the potatoes get cold. The advantage is that there is no waste.

2. Peeling before cooking. There is the maximum difference of texture between peeled and unpeeled surface when the potato is dry, but for someone with a little useful sight, washing the potato first prevents the white peeled surface becoming brown with soil, and the colour contrast between peeled and unpeeled areas is better. Actual peeling is best done with a potato peeler. One way of making sure of removing all the peel is to start at one end and peel round and round as when peeling an apple without breaking the peel. To make doubly sure a second layer can be peeled off, but this does mean a lot of the potato is wasted. Another method is to hold the potato in one hand with the forefinger at the top and the thumb at the bottom. Then peel downwards from top to bottom in overlapping strips, swivelling the potato round bit by bit. The small areas where the finger and thumb have held the potato are peeled at the end. The potato can be checked for eyes and bruises after peeling, but there is no foolproof way of being quite certain, other than seeking sighted help.

3. Serve potatoes in their jackets with a little chopped parsley and a knob of butter. This is the most nutritious way of serving potatoes. But it is necessary to be on friendly terms with the greengrocer and ask him to pick out only perfect potatoes. These only need to be scrubbed well before cooking. A pan scourer may be best for the job.

Some people check peeled potatoes by putting them into salty water. The peeled surface becomes slimy and the unpeeled parts feel rough.

Ways of boiling
Ideally cooker and sink should have only a working surface between them so that a pan of cooked vegetables does not have to be carried across the room for draining. Use a long-handled colander for straining to keep boiling water away from the hands. Otherwise a chip basket can be used to hold the vegetables inside the pan, and simply lifted out when they are done. There are also wire baskets with a finer mesh which are used for blanching vegetables for home freezing. These are available in different sizes from freezer centres and could be used for peas or anything else small. Cooks who are sufficiently experienced can also cook vegetables in very little water. Nutritionally this is by far the best method but it needs good hearing so as to know when the water is about to dry out.

A heavy-bottomed saucepan is essential for this last method of cooking. It is also better from the point of view of stability, especially on gas cookers which do not have a flat surface. Small saucepans, and especially milk saucepans which are wider at the top than at the bottom, are particularly prone to tip over on gas rings and should be avoided. However one way round this problem of small saucepans is to use a mat made of wire mesh to put under the pan. These Tomado stove mats are made in Holland and are intended to serve the same purpose as asbestos mats. (For details see p. 92.) Otherwise it is important to make sure the pan is square over the gas ring before lighting the gas, and the flame should never be too high for fear of burns if the flame curls around the sides of the pan; this is a waste of gas too.

One way of avoiding liquid boiling over is to use a large enough saucepan so that it is only necessary to half fill it. For boiling milk, some people like to use a milk-saver which is an ovenproof glass or aluminium disc which is put in the bottom of the milk pan. This disc rattles when the milk begins to boil. Milk-savers should be on sale at most hardware stores. It is a good idea to choose a milk pan with a lip at both sides so that either hand can be used for pouring. There is also a milk-saver pan specially designed to prevent milk boiling over, provided it is gently heated. (For details see page 89.)

Methods of frying
Frying is probably the most frightening way of cooking for a blind cook. But it should be possible to regain confidence in using a frying pan by starting off with something that requires very little fat or is not

likely to spurt. Fish fingers, fish cakes or potato cakes need no more than a dessertspoonful of fat per portion and are flat and easy to handle. It is important that the frying pan should have a heavy bottom and a firmly fixed handle. A light pan will be unstable, and will tend to buckle and burn food. For turning food over, a slice with a long flexible blade and a short handle is more likely to be of use than a short square blade with a long handle. Ideally the frying pan with a small quantity of fat should be placed on a ring or burner at the back of the cooker with its handle pointing to the side of the stove. After a few minutes the temperature of the fat can be tested by withdrawing the pan from the heat and putting the end of one fish finger in the pan. If the fat is hot enough there will be a gentle sizzling sound; if it is too hot the sizzling will be rather loud and silence indicates that the fat is not yet hot enough. Once the temperature is right, the fish fingers should be placed in the pan while it is away from the heat and then, using the fish slice, arranged in a block in line with the pan handle so that they can be easily located when it comes to turning over. Many blind people prefer to use tongs as it is easier to grip with these.

Using the oven
Many people prefer to avoid frying altogether and use their grill or the oven instead. But although this avoids the risks of being splashed with hot fat, it still involves getting food in casseroles or baking tins in and out of a hot oven. It is essential to wear oven gloves; if you can, find a pair that are large enough to go half-way up the forearm so that the delicate skin around the wrist is well protected. It is often possible to put food (e.g. a casserole) into a cold oven; but with cake mixes that have to be put into a hot oven it is probably easiest to cope safely if the tin is held in one hand only, and the other hand used to locate the shelf and guide the tin into its correct place. As oven cleaning is so difficult for a person who cannot see well, it is a wise precaution always to put a large roasting tin underneath any casserole dish to catch any drips. It is obviously best to use a large dish, only half full.

Making a cup of tea
This is the perennial problem of every newly blind person: 'How can I make myself a cup of tea?' This is the method first introduced to *In Touch* listeners by Jill Allen, another professional cook who had lost her sight but continued to look after her family unaided. Fill the

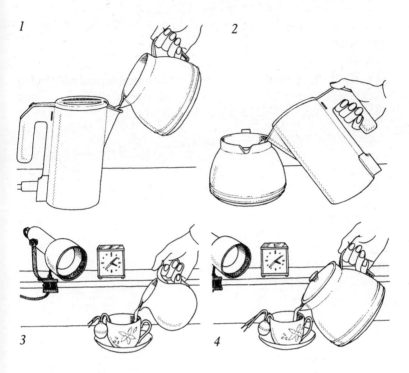

How to make a cup of tea

1 *Fill the teapot with cold water, and then pour into kettle to ensure that when boiling water is poured back into teapot, there will not be any surplus to overflow and scald the fingers.*

   Both the Redring Autoboil kettle and the Thermal teapot shown here are insulated so that they do not quickly get hot on the outside when filled with boiling water.

2 *Once the kettle has boiled, fill the teapot. Both the Redring kettle and the Thermal teapot have been recommended by blind users as easy to handle when pouring.*

3 *Use the liquid level indicator (long prong inside cup) when pouring the milk, and (4) reverse it (short prong inside) so that it will give an audible warning when cup is nearly full. For people with residual vision, it is important to have a good light over the working surface.*

teapot with cold water and then put this into the kettle: this ensures that when the boiling water from the kettle has to be poured back into the teapot there will not be any surplus to overflow and scald the fingers. While the kettle is boiling, warm the teapot by running hot water from the tap into it, then stand the teapot on the draining board, preferably on a dishcloth or a rubber mat to prevent it from slipping. Some people find it easier initially to make tea with teabags. Pour the boiling water in slowly, resting the spout of the kettle on the rim of the teapot. With practice both the changing sound of the water, and the difference in weight of the kettle, will be a guide to the fullness of the pot. Always put the kettle down at the back of the cooker to prevent it being accidentally knocked over. Pour milk into cups with short, sharp jerks of the wrist, rather than by trickling which is more difficult to control. One quick tilt should be enough. To pour from the teapot, rest the spout on the outer edge of the cup and put one finger of the left hand lightly over the opposite rim. With practice it is again possible to gauge by sound and time just how the cup is filling, but the left finger can feel the warmth of the tea fractionally before it reaches the top of the cup. There is no need to dip one's finger into the tea!

While most blind people can cope perfectly well with ordinary teapots and kettles, there are now some new models on the market which may be of particular use to blind people who are worried about scalding themselves. The thermal teapot has a surface which does not get hot, and the tea retains its heat for quite a long time. Jill Allen, who first recommended it to *In Touch* listeners, also said that she found the design of the pot, which has a very wide lid and a short spout, made it especially easy to fill and to pour from. It also has a removable strainer so that it is easy to clean. The teapot is made in several bright colours which may be helpful to partially sighted people (for details see page 92).

Another aid to blind tea makers is the unusually shaped Redring Autoboil kettle (see illustration page 101). This is a three-pint electric kettle with automatic switch-off and it retails at about £20, but in other respects it is quite different from the usual electric kettle. It is made of a plastic material which only warms up very slowly, so that immediately after the kettle has boiled it is barely warm to the touch, and it is therefore easy to handle. It does get warmer once it has stood for a while full of hot water, but it is never so hot as to scald anyone who touches it by accident. It looks rather like a vacuum jug, and the spout has a small lip which is useful to rest against the edge of a cup when pouring. Because the kettle is tall and narrow, with the electric element at the bottom, it will safely boil just one cupful of water at a time if required. It has a big, round, easy-to-grip handle. It is much lighter than ordinary metal kettles and so could be more practical for those with arthritic fingers. However, some people might find the lid rather stiff to remove if they did not wish to fill the kettle through its spout, and it is not very easy to feel the on/off switch (for details see page 88).

The liquid level indicator is a gadget which some blind people find a great boon when making tea. The longer wire goes on the inside of the cup to gauge how much milk to put in, then the gadget is reversed to put the shorter wire on the inside to give an audible indication when the cup is nearly full (for details see page 89).

Cookery books

While a limited number of cookery books have been produced in braille, large print and on tape, hardly any of these have been written with the needs of visually handicapped people in mind. The exception is the Clifton Spinney Cookery book which was compiled by staff at the RNIB's rehabilitation centre in Nottingham. This gives twenty-two recipes, most of them for oven dishes which can be put into a cold oven; but even this book does not always explain how a person with limited vision should carry out all the processes involved. There is both a large print and a tape version of Louise Davies' *Easy Cooking for One or Two*, which is available from Magna Print Books at *Magna House, Long Preston, North Yorkshire (tel. Long Preston (07294) 225)* for £3.50 and on tape from the *ADA Reading Service* at *12 Renhold Road, Wilden, Bedford (tel. Wilden (0234) 771693)*. To get the tape version of the book, which is slightly abridged, send two C60 cassettes. The ADA Reading Service can also supply extracts from Violet Stephenson's *Grow and Cook* (send three C60 cassettes for a copy of this). It is also possible to get a collection of 'cookery spots' done by Marguerite Patten for the *Soundaround* cassette magazine from *Nigel Verbeeck, 61 Church Road, Barnes, London SW13 (tel. 01-741 3332)*. There are two C60 cassettes which cost £1 each.

The *First and Second Jimmy Young Cookbooks* and the *Pennywise Cookbook*, published by the Milk Marketing Board, have been produced in Moon and are available from the National Library for the

103

Blind. The National Library also has published large-print versions of the *Grammar of Cookery* by Philip Harben, and the *Penguin Cookery Book* by Bee Nilson. These can be borrowed on request through the local public library.

A limited number of cookery books are available in braille from the National Library and the Scottish Braille Press. The Braille magazines *Home Help* and *Madam* published by the Scottish Braille Press also regularly include cookery recipes, selected from women's magazines. It is also possible to get cookery recipes transcribed into braille by one of the Braille Transcription Services (see pages 145–6 for details). The Voluntary Transcribers Group would be prepared, for a small additional charge, to transfer brailled recipes on to Braillon – this is a thin plastic sheet that can be wiped clean with a damp cloth. The various tape reading services would also be prepared to record recipes – or even complete cookery books – on to tape (see page 172 for details).

★ *Lay a wet cloth over the work surface when baking. Not only does it prevent utensils slipping about, but cleaning up afterwards is much easier. (Mrs. E. Fox, Bolton, Lancs.)*

★ *Put a rubber band halfway down on pots of marmalade, it's then easy to tell it from jam.*
(Maud Berry, Berkshire)

Using residual vision

Most 'blind' people have some sight. How useful it is depends on how well it is used, and the more it is used the more useful it is likely to become. Sitting in a dimly lit room with eyes half closed will not preserve sight; nor will denying oneself the pleasure of watching television, in order to avoid eyestrain, help. Indeed, ophthalmologists argue that eyestrain is a myth and that using remaining sight can neither strain nor damage the eyesight nor make it deteriorate more quickly. It is, however, much easier to listen to this excellent advice than to carry it out, for a number of factors combine to make it difficult to follow.

Many people when registered as blind feel they may be considered frauds if they admit to having some useful sight. The general public finds the idea of defective and distorted vision difficult to understand, and assumes that a person carrying a white stick is unable to see at all. Poor lighting in the home means that many visually handicapped people see less well than they should. A study of visually handicapped patients in 1978 suggested that for every ten patients who would be assessed as 'blind' in a well-lit hospital clinic, double that number would be so assessed if they were examined at home.[1] People think, mistakenly, that it is useless to seek professional help for failing sight. It is a sad fact that the patchy provision of low vision clinics and the scarcity of opticians with low vision expertise is a major reason why so many visually handicapped people function below their true visual capacity. It is estimated that only one third of registered blind and partially sighted people have a low vision assessment, and that it is likely that half of those who have not had the opportunity to try such aids would be likely to benefit from them.[2]

Residual vision
In this chapter, this phrase is used to describe the sight retained by a visually handicapped person who has been examined by an ophthal-

[1] *Visual Acuity at home and in eye clinics*: Silver, J. H., Gould, E. S., Irvine, D. and Cullinan, T. R. Trans. Ophthal. Soc. U.K. (1978) 98, p. 262.
[2] *The Provision of Low Vision Aids to the Visually Handicapped*: Silver, J. H., Gould, E. S. and Thomsitt, J. (1974) Trans. Ophthal. Soc. U.K. 94, pp. 310–9.

mologist and has been told 'nothing further can be done'. The examination is essential for without it those who are visually handicapped run the risk of solving their immediate problem by, for example, purchasing a magnifier when the eye condition causing the poor sight could be treated. In some cases, this could mean that they might be in danger of losing their sight completely, *whereas early diagnosis and treatment would save it*.

Residual vision varies from individual to individual, and for some people it even fluctuates during the day. All visually handicapped people 'see' differently. Many find it difficult to distinguish colours, especially the difference between red and green. Pastel colours may be seen as rather similar shades of grey but sharp contrasts in colours are likely to be noticed, though the colours seen may not be the true ones. Even two people who suffer from the same eye condition are unlikely to both have the same view of the world. However, some eye conditions primarily affect visual acuity (the ability to see clearly) and others mainly affect the visual field (the ability to see 'out of the corner' of one's eyes). Dividing eye conditions into these two categories is inevitably a rough and ready means of differentiation, but it does point the way to one of the most constructive means by which the visually handicapped can make the best use of their remaining sight. They are their own best experts when it comes to assessing what can or cannot be seen and the conditions needed to see, but if they can work out the rationale for this, they are well on the way towards using their remaining sight effectively. Of course, a professional with low vision expertise will be able to help them overcome the hurdles more easily, but in the absence of such help, there is much that individuals can do to help themselves.

Conditions affecting the visual field
The ability to see 'all round' – to see above, below and alongside the object being viewed is much more vital than is generally appreciated by people with good sight. It is this ability that enables us to locate ourselves, and identify objects, 'at a glance'. Glaucoma and retinitis pigmentosa are the most common causes of blindness which affect this visual function. In both conditions, peripheral (side) vision gradually deteriorates, and at an advanced stage this type of sight is aptly described as 'tunnel vision'.

When trying to use this restricted vision for the best effect, sufferers will increasingly have to 'scan'; that is, they will deliberately have to move their eyes and head to make the most effective use of the remaining field of vision. It will probably be easier to read narrow rather than wide columns of print. Sometimes they may find it easier to move the print across the line of vision in order to read it. Even when the loss is not too severe, keeping to the line and finding the next line may present problems. A mask (a piece of black card with a slot cut in it roughly the length and width of a line), or a pointer, may help. An optical means of helping increase this narrow field of vision is the field expander. This aid works on the same principle as the tiny glasses sometimes fitted on outside doors to enable the householder to see who is on the doorstep. Such aids are of particular value for distance or outdoor vision. Everything is reduced in size, so that the number of objects in view is increased. Their value can be appreciated by looking through the *wrong* end of a monocular distance telescope – the greater the magnification the greater the effect. Field expanders are available through low vision clinics but as yet their use is limited; nevertheless work on their development is continuing. Unfortunately ordinary magnifying aids for increasing the size of print are unlikely to help. They will make the sufferer see less, not more, as the limited field of vision will be filled with even fewer letters. An aid to enable a person with tunnel vision to 'see the whole page' rather than a tiny section of it has not yet been invented, though field expanders may be pointing the way.

Field loss does not, however, affect only the side vision. Field loss involving the right or left field of each eye is sometimes experienced by people who have suffered a stroke. This type of loss can be very incapacitating, especially as the sufferer may be in a frail state of health. As well as being unable to see obstacles on the affected side, difficulty will be experienced in reading, due to problems in finding the line and then keeping to it. This will be most pronounced if the right side of the field of each eye is lost, in which case special mirror spectacles may be required. A card mask or a pointer may help, or even a thumb placed at the beginning of the line being read.

Conditions affecting clarity of vision
Threading a needle, recognising a person's face or reading print are all examples of ways in which we put our central vision to use. If the central part of the retina has deteriorated, problems in distinguishing detail will be encountered. Macular degeneration, one of the most common causes of visual handicap in old age, has this effect. Side

vision usually remains unaffected, so at least the sufferer does not have severe problems in moving around.

To make the best use of this restricted vision will call for some ingenuity, for the aim will be to use side vision, where it exists, for some of the tasks previously carried out by central vision. The object to be distinguished will, therefore, most likely be seen more clearly when looking just to one side of it, rather than directly at it. The best side to look will vary from person to person; for some it may be to the right or left of the object, whilst for others it may be above or below. This new technique of looking takes time to learn but once mastered can be used to great advantage. The visually handicapped person can casually move alongside the person he wishes to see more clearly, relatives can make sure a cup of tea is placed on the 'good side' rather than immediately in front.

This type of vision is particularly likely to be helped by optical aids that magnify, ranging from simple hand-held magnifiers to electronic aids such as closed circuit television. Such aids will throw a larger image on the retina, and the bigger the image the greater chance it has to fall on the undamaged part and so be seen.

Clarity of vision is also blurred when field loss, mentioned earlier, is not confined to peripheral vision but affects areas of central vision. This results in 'patchy' vision, parts of the picture will be lost and the edges blurred, as can happen in diabetic retinopathy, and retinal detachment. Cataract also blurs vision, though the extent to which this handicaps an individual will depend on the size and position of the clouded area of the lens. Unhappily, it is not unusual for severely visually handicapped people to suffer from a combination of conditions, and so have both their peripheral field of vision and central vision affected, as happens when diabetic retinopathy is complicated by cataract, or macular degeneration by glaucoma. Even so, whilst there is some vision left a trial of low vision aids is worthwhile. The crucial factor is often not the amount of residual vision but the motivation of the patient.

Low vision aids
Motivation is all-important, because a low vision aid is quite different from the conventional spectacles which in the past have probably immediately enabled the patient to see everything clearly and easily. Low vision aids are job-specific and different ones are needed for

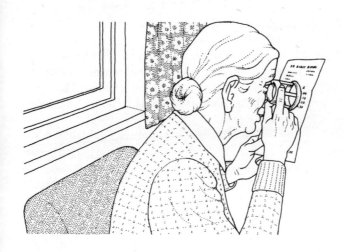

With high-powered magnifiers, it is important to hold the aid close to the eye, as well as the reading matter. This increases the field of view.

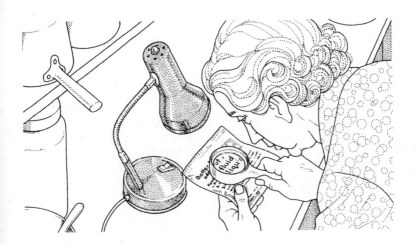

Low vision aids are not just for reading print

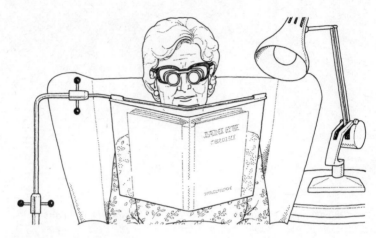

Spectacle magnifiers require the reading matter to be close to the eyes, and a book rest may help

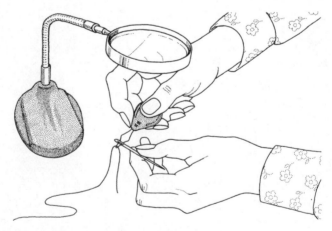

A stand magnifier leaves both hands free for work

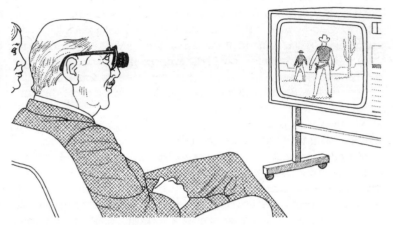

A monocular telescope clipped onto a spectacle frame can help some people to watch television

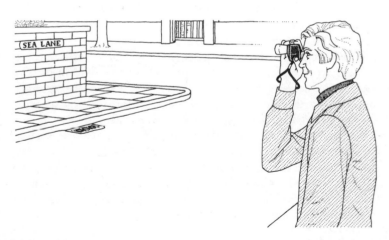

A monocular distance telescope can be used to read the number on a bus-stop, or the name of the street

different visual tasks. In addition, the use of vision aids for reading and writing will require holding things relatively close to the eyes. Spectacle magnifiers may be based on one of two designs – either a simple microscope or a telescope. Spectacle microscopes can be prescribed to enable people with very poor sight to read, but the print may have to be held only inches away from the spectacles. Even a simple high-powered hand or stand magnifier (see illustration on page 109) will need to be held close to the eye, and then the reading matter put close to the aid. Children accommodate without much difficulty to this reading position, but adults can find it much more difficult, though well worth the effort.

No doubt this is one of the reasons for the growing popularity of closed-circuit television, for with this aid very high magnification (up to 60 times) can be achieved and yet reading remains relatively relaxed and pleasurable as the user can sit comfortably two or three feet from the screen. Such systems do, however, reduce the field of view as the number of words displayed on the screen will decrease as the magnification is increased. CCTV consists of a vertically mounted television camera underneath which is a movable platform on which the reading matter is placed. Alongside, or above the camera, is a television monitor screen which shows the enlarged print either in black on a white ground or, as is often preferred, as white print on a black ground. CCTV can be used also for handwriting, and a typewriter can also be used underneath the camera.

For work where the reading matter must be at a distance, as happens when sitting at the piano or reading dials, intermediate or near vision telescopes may be prescribed. These are spectacle mounted but they do give a longer working distance than spectacle microscopes, albeit at the price of a restricted field.

A range of telescopes can be obtained for distance use, such as identifying bus stops or watching television. These vary from a monocular clip-on version which can be attached to ordinary spectacles if the user has useful vision in one eye, to spectacle mounted binoculars (such as the sportscopes seen at race meetings) and tiny hand-held monoculars (see illustrations on page 111).

Obtaining a low vision aid
It will be apparent that, because of the wide range of low vision aids and the differing needs of patients, professional help should be sought if possible so that the right aid is found. Low vision aids (except

CCTV) can be prescribed through the Hospital Eye Service, generally at low vision clinics attached to Eye Hospitals or University Ophthalmic Optics departments. Patients need to be referred by an ophthalmologist. Low vision aids can also be purchased privately, but again a referral from an ophthalmologist will be needed by all reputable low vision practitioners. Hospital clinics and private practitioners are unevenly distributed throughout the country, but details can be obtained from *Mrs V. Scarr, FSMC, FBOA, Adviser on Visual Impairment at the Disabled Living Foundation (tel. 01-602 2491, Wednesdays only, 10 am – 2 pm).*

The Association of Optical Practitioners, Bridge House, 233-4 Blackfriars Road, London, SE1 8NW (tel. 01-261 9661) will also refer enquirers to opticians able to supply low vision aids.

Closed-circuit television is not supplied through the National Health Service, though sets are likely to be on show at low vision clinics. It may be supplied under the Aids to Employment Scheme (see page 50) or by LEAs for educational purposes. CCTV can be purchased (prices range from £800 – £1,500) from three manufacturers: *John Heathcote and Co. Ltd, Focus Division, Tiverton, Devon (tel. Tiverton (0884) 254949), Alphamed Ltd, 61 Beechtree Avenue, Marlow Bottom, Buckinghamshire SL7 3NH (tel. Marlow (06284) 71370)* and *Wormald International Sensory Aids Ltd, 7 Musters Road, West Bridgeford, Nottingham (tel. Nottingham (0602) 865995/6)*, or through private low vision practitioners, such as *C. Davis Keeler Ltd, 21/7 Marylebone Lane, London W1M 6DS (tel. 01-935 8512)* who distribute Magna-vision.

Self-help and low vision aids
Because of the shortage of professional expertise, there is an increasing number of lay sources of help. The Partially Sighted Society has demonstration kits of aids which can be examined at some of their branches, and selections of aids can be found at many Aids Centres and at rehabilitation centres. Some social services departments stock a range of magnifiers, as do a number of voluntary societies for the blind. Some voluntary societies, including the Royal National Institute for the Blind, have demonstration closed-circuit television sets. CCTV is also to be found in a number of libraries; fuller details can be obtained from the Development Officer at the Library Association.

The Disabled Living Foundation has a permanent exhibition of low vision aids and has a training kit which can be hired. The kit is designed for professional use only (medical and paramedical) and includes a very wide selection of aids from the most sophisticated prescription aid down to the simplest magnifier.

Choosing a simple magnifier: Even selecting a simple magnifier has traps for the unwary. Large size and high magnification never go together, and a sheet which magnifies a whole page gives a very low magnification indeed. It is helpful if the relative or friend trying to assist the visually handicapped person unable to get professional advice, tries to establish the magnification needed to enable print to be read. The chart on pages 284–7 can be used to give this guidance. The visually handicapped person should sit in a good light, with reading spectacles if worn, and decide which is the smallest line of print that can be read correctly. A considerable effort may be required to distinguish the print and it may only be possible to correctly identify the individual letters of each word rather than whole words on the line. Underneath that line is the approximate magnification required to enable ordinary newsprint to be read. A magnifier of that strength should be sought.

It is not enough, however, just to consider magnification when making a choice. A hand magnifier should be light and easy to hold if the purchaser intends to read with it, for it will have to be held steady at the correct focus for long periods. If there is a hand tremor, a magnifier on a stand which is pushed along the page would be a better choice. Flat field magnifiers which look like glass paperweights are often useful as they focus a great deal of light on the text and can be easily pushed along the line. Magnifiers which look like torches, as they have a light incorporated in them, can be obtained in a variety of strengths and because of their built-in illumination may solve problems which would normally be resolved only by stronger – and therefore smaller – magnifiers.

Apart from high street opticians' shops, magnifiers can be purchased in places as diverse as supermarkets, garages, and photographic shops. The magnification is generally marked on the box or on the magnifier itself (2x, 5x, 7x etc.) Sometimes, instead, the power is expressed in dioptres. Divide the number of dioptres by four to establish the magnifying strength.

Useful catalogues which indicate the range of simple magnifiers on sale include those issued by *Combined Optical Industries, 200 Bath Road, Slough SL1 4DW (tel. Slough (0753) 21292), Newbould and*

Bulford, Enbeeco House, Carlton Park, Saxmundham, Suffolk IP17 2NL, and *Edward Marcus, 7 Moorfields, London EC2Y 9AE.*

Lighting

Most visually handicapped see better if they can work in a good light. Elderly people in general need more light than they did in their younger days to see detail, and this applies equally to the elderly with a visual handicap. The level of lighting in their homes should be much better than average, and the light levels between rooms and corridors roughly the same. To come out of a brightly lit bathroom on to a stairway or landing lit by one 60-watt bulb can be very dangerous. On the other hand, some visually handicapped people are very sensitive to light, especially those suffering from retinitis pigmentosa, albinism or cataract, and are quick to point out that they find bright lights painful and that they see very badly on sunny days. It is important here to distinguish between sensitivity to light and sensitivity to glare. People suffering from cataract may well see very badly in sunshine, whilst seeing without difficulty under other conditions (the effect is the same as that experienced by the car driver who can see through his dirty windscreen until he drives into the setting sun). This is because the cataract makes them very susceptible indeed to dazzle. They are still likely to see better in good lighting as long as the sources of light are carefully shaded, the surfaces on which the light shines are not too shiny and reflective and – for close work – the lighting is directed on to the task in hand from behind. Unfortunately, little research has been carried out to discover the lighting levels required by people suffering from different eye pathologies to enable them to perform specific visual tasks, but a common-sense rule is that those people who find their sight markedly poorer in artificial light than in daylight, or who dislikes dark, dull days for the same reason, should immediately try to improve the level of their lighting.

Improving lighting levels

A high level of illumination does not necessarily mean incurring great expense. Natural daylight is a very strong source of light, and completely free. Curtains should, therefore, be pulled well back. Even net curtains can exclude a great deal of light. Furniture should be moved, if necessary, to take advantage of the daylight. Anyone with poor sight who is bedridden is likely to see better if the bed does *not* face the only

115

window in the room but is set at an angle to it. Walls painted with a light-coloured matt emulsion paint reflect much more light than a sombre wallpaper and a fresh coat of white emulsion paint can lighten a room to an extent which has to be experienced to be believed. When these simple alterations have been made, it is then a good idea to consider the electrical fittings.

There are many light fittings on the market which visually handicapped people would find useful, such as spot lights, clip-on-lights, and concealed lighting, but many will find their needs are met just by having powerful light bulbs in the conventional pendant ceiling fitting. Unless the ceiling is very high, a pendant light fitted with a simple white shade, wider at the bottom than the top, and equipped with a 100-watt or 150-watt pearl bulb should give sufficient general light in the average sitting room. Fluorescent lights are also well worth considering for living rooms as well as for kitchens. The expense of their installation is offset to some extent by the fact that they use less electricity than conventional lights and the tubes last a very long time indeed. De luxe white tubes give a light similar in colour to ordinary household lighting.

For close work, good general lighting needs to be supplemented by direct light from an adjustable lamp, angled so that the light falls on the work, ideally from a point behind the individual. It is important to remember that the distance between the lamp and the object to be illuminated is crucial. Halving the distance will quadruple the amount of light. It is for this reason that a standard lamp alongside a low armchair rarely gives a visually handicapped person a sufficiently high level of illumination for reading; the distance between lamp and book is too great.

When choosing an adjustable lamp it is wise to choose one with a good stable base, but not so heavy that it will be difficult to move. The on/off switch should be easy to reach and find, preferably on the base. It should be easy to adjust and the shade should totally screen the light bulb from the eyes whilst directing the light on the work in hand. The ideal lamp does not yet exist, but in 1981 the Lighting Division of the Chartered Institute of Building Services and the Partially Sighted Society were working together to establish a performance specification for an effective reading lamp for people with poor sight. In the meantime, British Home Stores have a wide range of adjustable lamps taking 60-watt light bulbs. This wattage is usually sufficient if the lamp can be brought close to the work. Table lamps taking 100-watt bulbs, which can be helpful for people needing a greater distance between lamp and task, are more difficult to find, but are manufactured by *Anglepoise Ltd, Enfield Industrial Estate, Unit 51, Redditch, Worcester (tel. Redditch (0527) 63771)* and *Thousand-and-One Lamps Ltd, 108 Bromley Road, London SE6 2UX (tel. 01-698 7238)*.

Advice on lighting

The Partially Sighted Society is particularly concerned with lighting and has a building and environmental consultancy service which can advise on lighting design and engineering, decor, and architecture. Their publication *Light for Low Vision* (inkprint and cassette) is a valuable source of information both for individuals wishing to improve their home lighting and for professionals involved in building schemes. Help and advice should also be available through local social services departments. A spokesman for the Department of Health and Social Security has stated that 'visually handicapped people should consult their social services department under the terms of the Chronically Sick and Disabled Persons Act 1970 if they feel that improved lighting is needed. If the social services department agree the provision is necessary, they will make all the arrangements themselves. They may require the person concerned to meet the cost or to make a contribution towards it.'

Protection from glare

Usually it is light that comes from above or from the side that is most troublesome. A hat with a brim, a sunvisor on a fabric band or cap, a peaked cap like those worn by baseball players (which have the bonus of also giving protection to the face) or a traditional green eyeshade may well be both the best and simplest solution. Sportswear shops, chemists and swimwear sections of departmental stores often stock them. In cases of difficulty, sunvisors on a fabric band can be obtained through *Lillywhites Mail Order, Lillywhites Ltd, Piccadilly Circus, London SW1 (tel. 01-930 3181)* and blue or green plastic shades on an adjustable elastic band, from *Solport Brothers Ltd, Portia House, Goring Street, Goring-by-Sea, Worthing, Sussex BN12 5AD (tel. Worthing (0903) 44861)*.

This simple solution is to be preferred to using sunglasses out of doors, which inevitably cut down the light reaching the eyes – the very light the eyes need to function as well as possible. However, some visually handicapped people do complain of great difficulty in seeing

in brightly lit surroundings. Tinted lenses, some of which are graduated, the darkest tint being at the top, can be prescribed through the
National Health Service when there is a real medical need for them. In
1979, fifty people suffering from retinitis pigmentosa tried out a range
of different sunglasses and from this limited survey the following
guidelines emerged which other visually handicapped people might
find useful when choosing sunglasses.[1]

If you normally wear glasses:

1 Ask your optician to show you brown tints first, then the grey or
the green.

2 If in doubt, select the lighter tint (after all, you spend most of your
life indoors) and get an industrial protective shield to wear over your
spectacles outdoors.

3 If you do not have a very strong prescription, have it made up in a
palish solid tint. The lens can be coated in a darker tint later.

4 If you are one of the people who wants things even darker, go for a
spectacle lens in one colour and a shield in another.

5 Avoid rimless and metal frames unless they can be fitted close to
the eye.

If you do not wear glasses:

1 Try an industrial protective spectacle first.

2 Look for wrap-around sun spectacles with brown, grey or green
lenses.

3 It is well worth having a look at Reactolite Rapide or Polarmatic
lenses, but do try them outdoors first if at all possible.

The industrial protective shields mentioned can be obtained from
*Chubb Panorama Ltd, Industrial Estate, Evans Place, Bognor Regis,
W. Sussex PO22 9RH (tel. 0243 828911)*, model EM 673, £1.60.

Visual clues

The onset of severe visual handicap is generally in middle or late life.
Visually handicapped people will, therefore, be faced with the almost
irresistible temptation of constantly comparing their present sight
with that which they previously enjoyed. This is natural enough in the
early days, but it is a fact that continued constant reiteration of what
cannot be seen is a certain way of losing friends and alienating people.

[1] Silver, J. *Tinted Lenses*: Bulletin 12, Autumn 1979. British Retinitis Pigmentosa
Society.

It also prevents the visually handicapped person from making the best use of the sight that is retained. Difficult though it may be to discern it, there is, amidst the haze of blurred vision, one priceless asset: clear visual memories. In other words, the completed jigsaw pattern has already been seen so that now, when some of the pieces are missing or distorted, there is still the potential of reconstructing the whole in the mind's eye. But as many visual 'clues' as possible will be needed – those distinctive jigsaw shapes that when slotted into the pattern suddenly make all the hitherto meaningless pieces spring to life.

Unfortunately, there is no list of visual clues that all visually handicapped people find helpful; as we have seen, no two people have the same residual vision. Therefore, only the individual can decide what clues are needed, and under what conditions. Clues are, however, more likely to be identified when lighting is adequate, when they are brightly coloured – orange, yellow, and light green are generally especially helpful – and when their colour and shape contrast with the surroundings. The gross characteristics of objects are more likely to yield clues than the fine ones; the dark mound on the chair which elongates slowly is more likely to be a cat than a cushion – or even a dog! Visual clues can also be reinforced by data from other senses, so that clues provided by sight, hearing and touch can combine to enable a person to move confidently and act decisively.

Relatives and friends can help in identifying visual clues by noticing which colours are seen best and using them unobtrusively to denote hazards. When shopping, they can look for items in colours which are known to be helpful; a simple example is the brightly coloured plastic beaker holder which enables an otherwise almost invisible glass of water to be seen on the bedside table. But much must be left to the visually handicapped person's own inventiveness and ingenuity. Each must decide if a red plate shows up the food outlined against it, whether the antimacassar draped over the arm of an easy chair will prevent a collision with it. If print can no longer be read, the visually handicapped person may well feel that visual clues are of little use, for example in sorting out correspondence; this is, however, far from being the case. The shape and colour of an envelope can often indicate its origin whilst the heavy black type (On Her Majesty's Service), even though it appears only as a blur, tells its own story. Similarly, in the supermarket, you do not need to be able to read 'Kellogg's Cornflakes' in order to identify the correct packet. The design on the packet will indicate the brand, as the manufacturers intended. To the visually handicapped person the design may be merely a yellow splodge, with black print at the left and topped by red, but this will give sufficient information, once it has been recognised.

Yet this is only the beginning of achievement for this group of individuals. If there is residual vision present, then, for many people, meaningful reading is an attainable goal. In order to read, however, the reading techniques used by the normally sighted must be discarded. It is no longer possible to read in a conventional way – by looking at whole words and phrases, taking them in and comprehending their meaning instantly. It is, however, possible in most cases, with the help of a suitable aid, to see the individual letters of each word. Words can, therefore, be built up as one goes along rather than by seeing them as they are printed – as whole units. Reading by this technique is slower than by traditional methods, particularly at first, but at least it does enable reading to be carried out. It is one of the important means by which the visually handicapped can remain independent.

The emphasis that this chapter has given to the use of residual vision is one of the new and most exciting developments in work with the visually handicapped. In recent years the Research Centre for the Education of the Visually Handicapped (Faculty of Education, Birmingham University) and the Schools Council have worked together on a Visual Perception Training Project. As a result, in 1979 the *Look and Think* diagnostic kit and teacher's handbook were published. The kit is no longer available, but it has been replaced by the *Look and Think Teachers' File*. The File gives advice on the construction of the teaching materials mentioned in the handbook which are not commercially available and advises on the adaptation of published material for particular visual perception training purposes. Both the *Teachers' Handbook* and the *Teachers' File* can be purchased from the RNIB (Education Department). Visual perception training for adults is still in its early stages, with much of the development work being carried out at Torquay Rehabilitation Centre (see page 45) and at low vision clinics attached to major Eye Hospitals and University Ophthalmic Optics Departments.

Further reading
Aids to Vision: G. Marshall (30p from Waterside, The Green, Long Itchington, Rugby.)

Subnormal Vision: R. Greenhalgh. The Partially Sighted Society
Light for Low Vision: Proceedings of the Symposium held at University College, London, 4.4.1978. The Partially Sighted Society

I was always losing my tools around the garden; my trowel and hand-fork being the worst offenders. Then I had the bright idea – in more ways than one – of painting the handles of my garden tools in bright yellow. Now I can spot them more easily and save myself no end of time searching for them.
(Rosie Richardson, Darlington)

Shiny door knobs which reflect the light can serve as useful clues to anyone with even a little residual sight and help them to find their way around the room.
(Mr. V. Sheppard, Leicester)

A loop of fairly thick white string on the keys to cupboards and drawers shows up well on dark furniture and if the key falls out it can be more easily found. My white doors have large black handles, so I loop the string round the handles, and if the keys falls out, it hangs there and does not fall to the ground.
(D.E. Howes, Horley)

It can be very difficult to see electric flexes that trail across the floor. White polystyrene moulding, used by decorators, can be used to cover them so that they are much more clearly visible.
(Frances Swinn, Gainsborough, Lincs.)

10 Getting around

If newly blind people are to learn to move about again freely, both they and the people they live with have some important adjustments to make. Some are practical, such as the suggestions listed below but, overriding everything else, is the need to establish rather than diminish a blind person's self-confidence, especially in ability to do things. The natural instinct of any close relative or friend is to help by doing as much as possible for a newly-blinded person, but it is probably kinder to encourage them to do as much as possible for themselves.

In the home
Most people know the layout of their homes pretty well, and with practice can remember where various pieces of furniture are in a room, and learn how to avoid bumping into them. The first and most important lesson to learn in a family with a blind member, is always to put things back where they belong. A wastepaper basket in the middle of the floor, a vacuum cleaner left in a passageway or, worse, halfway up the stairs, or even a chair or coffee table put into a different position, can not only trip and injure a blind person, but severely shake his or her confidence. Never leave doors half open; it can be a very painful experience to walk into the side of a door. Blind people rarely need to have any alterations to the interior of houses for their safety. The exceptions are the very elderly, who may already have difficulties in movement; and some suggestions to help them are listed in Chapter 18, *Help for the elderly*. But if anyone in a family has severely restricted vision, it is worth having a general look at each room for likely sources of accident or injury.

Hall and passageway
To help a person with restricted vision, it is important to put in a high wattage bulb, particularly where there are steps and stairs. Check the banisters for safety. Do they go on right to the end of the steps? Quite a number, particularly in older houses, have a nasty trick of ending at the step before last. Any holes in stair covering are, of course, very dangerous for a blind person. If coat hooks or hat pegs protrude from the wall at or below face level, raise them a few inches or, if they cannot be moved, cover them with soft padding.

Sitting room and dining room

Nobody wants to rearrange his or her home radically; and a person who has suffered loss of sight may find it comforting that furniture is not changed around too much. It is helpful if the blind person's favourite chair is easily accessible from the door – so that it can be confidently approached without the risk of knocking into other objects on the way. It is important for a blind person to have a clear path; but there is no need to get obsessive about tidying everything away. It is easier if dining chairs are pushed under the table, rather than left standing in different positions on the floor; and floor-standing ornaments, such as tall vases, are a bit of a menace to someone who cannot see. If there are frail knick-knacks, keep them towards the back of a shelf or cupboard, rather than near the edge, where an inadvertent hand movement can knock them flying.

Bedroom

This usually presents few problems. Most people have no difficulty in finding their way around their own bedroom – though especially with an elderly person, the one route through the house which will cause particular anxiety is that from bedroom to toilet. If someone is not very independent when moving around, it might be worth considering the possibilities of changing the bedroom for one nearer the toilet.

Kitchen

Chapter 7, *In the kitchen*, has suggestions for ways in which the visually handicapped cook can cope efficiently.

Moving about safely

The hazards of moving about outside the house are infinitely greater than those inside, and there is relatively little a blind person can do to remove hazards. But the increasing encroachment of bicycles, shop displays and parked cars on pavements inspired the National Federation of the Blind to start a 'Give us Back our Pavements' campaign in 1979. This campaign is still going on, with increasing backing from organisations such as Age Concern and the Pedestrians Association. Full details from *Mrs Jill Allen, 59 Silversea Drive, Westcliff on Sea, Essex (tel. Southend (0702) 74059)*.

The whole technique of teaching a blind person to move about safely is still relatively new. The National Mobility Centre in

Birmingham, which was established in 1966, is responsible for the training of instructors (known as mobility officers) who teach blind people ways of moving about safely and effectively both indoors and out, using a variety of aids and techniques. At the time of writing, about seventy local authorities have appointed mobility officers; and blind people covered by these authorities can apply to the social services department for instruction in mobility. Tuition is usually on an individual basis and, as more instructors are trained, should become more generally available.

Techniques of mobility
Instinctively an untrained blind person holds an arm out straight ahead to feel the way. But this, in fact, is not a very effective technique, as it gives very little protection, and offers limited information about what lies ahead on only one side of the body. Mobility experts teach blind people various techniques for protecting themselves. The most generally useful indoor position is that in which one arm is raised to shoulder level, and then the elbow is bent to bring the forearm about twelve inches in front of the face. A totally blind person can check if this hand is in line with the face by blowing to find out if he or she can feel their own breath on the back of the hand. The palm of the hand should be facing outwards and the fingers extended so that their tips are in line with the opposite shoulder (see illustration). The use of this technique means that the face and head are protected – and while it is no guarantee against bumps, it is much less painful to knock into something with the palm of one's hand than with one's face. The other hand can be used to trail a wall or other guideline. The back of the hand should be in contact with the wall and the fingers lightly curled to avoid jamming them in openings.

A similar technique should be used by a blind person when bending down, because it is very easy to get a nasty blow from the edge of a chair or some other object. Before bending, the blind person should spread the fingers of one hand fan-like about six inches to eight inches in front of the face; it is much safer to squat bending the knees than to bend forward from the waist.

Another way in which mobility instructors can help is by showing blind people how to make the best possible use of their other senses. As they lose their sight, many people instinctively learn to get information from their ears or their sense of smell; others can learn this with expert advice. Often a simple suggestion may help. A blind

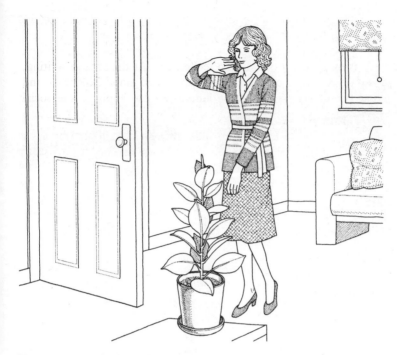

How to protect the face when moving about indoors; but doors should never be left half-open in any household that includes a blind person.

person who easily loses the sense of direction, even at home, can use the sound of a clock ticking on a mantelpiece or a portable radio placed on a table to act as a sound beacon to help find the way around.

One of the mobility officers' main jobs is to teach visually handicapped people how to use white sticks effectively. A blind person with a white stick is a familiar sight to most people, but it is not generally appreciated that there is quite a range of types of sticks (or canes as they are professionally called) intended for use in different ways. All types are available through the RNIB. The cheapest, and best known, is the 'symbol cane', which is made of sections of light metal tubing, joined together by an elastic cord. These canes are very light, and can be easily folded to fit into a handbag or a pocket. As their name implies, the symbol canes are intended as a signal to others that their user is visually handicapped. They are also intended as a probe or bumper, providing warning of obstacles ahead but they are not strong enough to give support. Those who need a white stick they

125

can lean on can buy a crook-handled white wooden walking stick from the RNIB. No special technique is needed to make use of either of these white sticks but more and more visually handicapped people are being trained by mobility officers to use another type of white stick, known as the 'long cane'.

This technique, pioneered in the United States, was first introduced here in the mid-1960s. The long cane is a light-weight aluminium tube with a crook handle and a special rubber grip at the top. Its length is tailored to the user's height and stride. It usually reaches to mid-chest height when held upright. The user holds the stick in front of the body at an angle of about thirty degrees to the ground, and moves it from side to side in an arc roughly the width of the body to check the ground ahead. The cane is swung to the left as the user steps out with the right foot, and vice versa (see illustration).

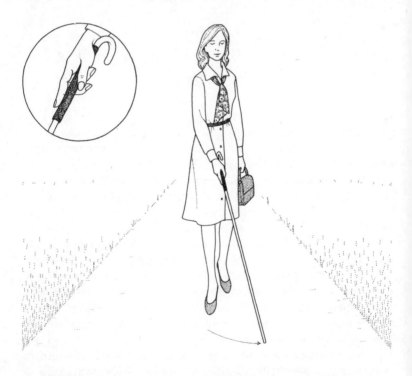

The long cane technique: the cane is swung to the left as the user steps out with her right foot. The long cane grip (top left)

Once trained, the user can walk quickly and confidently as proper use of the long cane technique gives warning of all obstacles in the way. This technique, which with practice becomes automatic, does require skilled training; but because of the shortage of mobility officers instruction is not always available. Training takes between three and four months of regular daily tuition, usually done from a person's own home.

Where training in the long cane technique is not locally available, suitable people may be referred to a residential rehabilitation course at one of the RNIB's centres, at which long cane training is given as well as instruction in other skills, such as braille and typing. 'Guide canes', which are a tougher version of the symbol cane, are also available from the RNIB in lengths ranging from 85 cms to 115 cms. No special training is needed to use these but it is possible, particularly with the larger guide canes, to use a modified version of the long cane technique; and sometimes elderly people find that their mobility needs are adequately met by this training. However, these guide canes do not have the special rubber grip of the long canes, so it may not be so easy to maintain the special hand position essential to carry out this tech nique correctly and effectively.

Both the guide canes and the long canes are fitted with replaceable tips, made of aluminium, rubber, metal or nylon. Replacement tips are available free from the RNIB and as each type of tip seems to have its own merits, it might be as well for each cane user to experiment and see which is the most suitable (see illustration on page 127).

All long canes are fitted with reflectorised tape and other white canes can on request be fitted with strips of reflecting tape; this is particularly useful for people in unlit country districts, where motorists rely on headlights. This tape is not, however, likely to give reflection in built-up areas with street lighting (see page 65 for suggestions about clothing for blind pedestrians).

Information about the availability of mobility training can be obtained in the first place from local authorities' social services departments. The National Mobility Centre does not train individual blind people, but is able to give information about training facilities in various parts of the country.

Mobility officers also have their own professional body, the National Association of Orientation and Mobility Instructors, which might be able to put people in touch with mobility instructors in their own area. Write to *Mrs Astrid Klemz, 31 Tennyson Road, Hutton,*

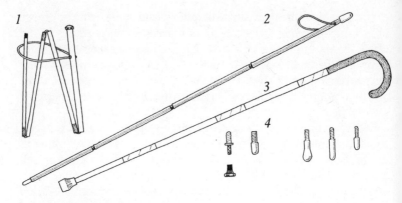

1 *The symbol cane folds up easily*
2 *The guide cane (which can also be folded up into four sections*
3 *White support stick with bands of reflective tape for extra protection at night, and a rubber tip for stability*
4 *A selection of tips for use with long canes and guide canes*

Brentwood, Essex CM13 2SJ, for contacts in the southern part of Britain, or to *Miss P. B. Airey, 2 Warren Terrace, Gilstead, Bingley, West Yorkshire BD16 3LD* for the north.

Guide dogs
A mobility aid which is familiar to many members of the public is the guide dog. There are at the moment about 2,700 guide dog owners in the country. Only registered blind people are eligible to apply for a guide dog, and the Guide Dogs for the Blind Association reserves the right to reject applicants without giving reasons for its decision. In general, however, guide dogs are recommended for fit and active people, over the age of 17, who can show evidence that they will do a regular amount of daily travelling. The majority of guide dog owners are blind people of working age, but older people who take regular exercise have also been accepted for training with a dog. The Association is, understandably, anxious to convince itself that a potential guide dog owner is likely to be going out regularly, even if only on short local trips to the shops, and not primarily wanting a dog just for companionship without making use of its special training. Applications can be made direct to the Guide Dogs for the Blind Association,

either by the blind person or by a relative, friend, or social worker on their behalf. A doctor's certificate of fitness will be required, and the local blind welfare authority will also be asked to endorse the application if they have not made the original request. The applicant will be interviewed at home by the representative of the Guide Dogs for the Blind Association, both to assess what is needed and to decide what kind of dog would be most suitable, and also to see whether the home conditions are suitable for a guide dog. The Association would want to be assured that there are adequate facilities for exercising a dog in the neighbourhood and that the applicant is aware of the responsibility involved in dog-ownership.

Once accepted, there is usually a waiting period of up to eighteen months. Training is residential and carried out at one of the five centres of the Association, at Exeter, Leamington Spa, Bolton, Wokingham and Forfar; it usually takes four weeks. In 1972, the Association decided to ask each blind person to pay a token 50p towards the cost of the dog and £1 a week board and lodgings towards the cost of their training course. Another factor that must be taken into consideration is the cost of keeping the dog. As guide dogs are invariably large – most frequently Labradors, golden retrievers or Alsatians – cost of feeding can be £3 a week. The Association pays a dog maintenance allowance of 25p a day to all guide dog owners, but in cases of financial difficulties it may be possible to get a grant either from the Association or a local welfare association. All guide dogs are registered with a vet, and each dog gets a free check-up twice a year. In fact many vets do not charge at all for their services to guide dogs, but if a guide dog owner is faced with veterinary bills that he or she cannot afford, the Association would consider helping to pay them.

Sonic aids
Other developments in recent years have been the various electronic mobility aids. The first of these, the ultrasonic torch, was invented by Dr (now Professor) Leslie Kay at Birmingham University in the early 1960s. The torch was held in the hand and transmitted a beam of high frequency sound ahead of the blind user, and some of this sound was reflected back by obstacles in the traveller's path, even when they were as much as twelve – or even twenty – feet away. The distance of the obstacles was indicated by the pitch of a note heard through an earpiece. A number of people were trained to use it, but although some were – and remained – enthusiastic about its value, many found

the signals difficult to interpret and the torch difficult to carry particularly if they also needed a cane. Also the torch did not indicate down kerbs with any degree of reliability.

Soon after developing the ultrasonic torch, Professor Kay took up a post in New Zealand and there he worked for some years on the development of sonic spectacles which, like the torch, worked on the 'bat' principle of reflected sound, but had the advantage that they freed the wearer's hands to use other mobility aids. This idea has been tested and refined for a number of years and, in 1977, the Sonicguide, a binaural aid, was first made available in this country.

The Sonicguide looks like a conventional pair of spectacles, but the centre of the frame incorporates a transmitter which radiates ultrasound (high frequency sound inaudible to the human ear) in front of the wearer. When the ultrasound hits an obstruction such as a car, a person or a lamp-post, it is reflected to the aid and received by two microphones in the spectacle frame. The microphones transform these reflected signals into electrical signals which are converted into audible sounds by two small earphones in the arms of the spectacle frame. Careful training is needed before a visually handicapped person can learn to use the Sonicguide, which, its makers claim, can locate and identify objects up to a distance of approximately five metres. The Sonicguide is expensive, and costs about £1,100. It is not intended to replace other mobility aids such as a long cane or guide dog, but to augment the rather limited information a blind person otherwise has about the environment. Full information about the Sonicguide and training facilities in Britain from Simon Foreacre at Wormald International Sensory Aids Ltd.

Wormald are also the makers of the Mowat Sensor, a hand-held tactile device intended to be used as a secondary aid to supplement other mobility aids such as a cane or guide dog. It was invented by a New Zealander, Geoff Mowat. The sensor employs high frequency sound to detect objects within a narrow beam (15 degrees) and at a range of up to 4 metres; if an object is present it vibrates, making it particularly valuable to a deaf-blind user. It is small enough to go into a pocket or handbag and as it does not emit any sound a blind person should be able to use it unobtrusively in public. The makers claim that it is sensitive enough to detect a coin lying flat on a table, but anticipate that its main value will be to help locate doorways, gaps between parked cars or find objects such as a letter box. It is not cheap – about £200 – and the user will need to have several hours training.

Full details from Simon Foreacre, Wormald International Sensory Aids Ltd.

Another electronic mobility aid has been produced by Dr Tony Heyes of the Blind Mobility Research Unit at Nottingham University. The Nottingham Obstacle Detector (NOD) is a hand-held ultrasonic aid – about the size of a large torch – which is designed to detect obstacles within 2.4 metres (8 feet) from the aid. The NOD's output comprises the eight notes of the musical scale, so that as a user approaches an obstacle he hears the descending notes of the scale giving an approximate indication of its actual distance. The NOD costs about £120. The Blind Mobility Research Unit has also devised the Sonic Pathfinder, a spectacle-worn obstacle detector, which like NOD represents the distance of an obstacle in terms of the eight notes of the musical scale. A limited number of the Pathfinders have been made, and according to Dr Heyes, the blind people who have been evaluating them have needed little training in their use and found them very acceptable. Full details of both devices from *Dr A. D. Heyes, Blind Mobility Research Unit, Department of Psychology, University of Nottingham, University Park, Nottingham NG7 2RD (tel. Nottingham (0602) 56101).*

Some years ago when mobility experts considered that the original sonic torch had been superseded, one enthusiastic blind user, Ernie Benham, set up Vol-Staic, a centre to encourage other people who wanted to use sonic aids. The original Kay torch is now being phased out, but is being replaced by Guidepath Mark 1, an obstacle detector which gives both audible and vibratory signals. Mr Benham states that he will supply the Guidepath on a month's free trial to all blind people who think they can make use of it; and if they can then prove that they are able to profit by it, Vol-Staic, which is a charity, will supply the equipment on permanent free loan under a sponsorship scheme. Vol-Staic also supplies chest- and wrist-mounted models of the original Kay torch (price £60) and will also supply sonic aid equipment suitable for use by blind people confined to a wheelchair. Full details from *E. H. Benham, Vol-Staic (Voluntary Sonic Travel Aid Instruction Centre for the Blind) 22 West Way, Lancing, West Sussex BN15 8LX (tel. Lancing (090 63) 64474).*

In addition to knowing whether or not one is likely to encounter an obstacle when moving about, it is also infuriating for a blind person to have to search a space, like a garden or even a large room, for a particular object. Two devices have been designed to overcome this.

The Homer is a pocket-sized sonic device which, when switched on, remains silent until triggered by a hand-clap or any sudden noise. It then emits a three-second clearly audible signal. This device could for example be left by a chair or lawn-mower in the garden so that a blind person can easily find them again. It can be hung from a door knob in a corridor full of identical doors to locate an office. The Homer is made in a sheltered workshop for disabled people, and costs £6.33 from *Castleham Industries, Collett Close, St Leonards on Sea, Sussex (tel. Hastings (0424) 53629)*.

The sound beacon obtainable from the RNIB is a similar device, which gives off sounds that can vary from a loud continuous whistle to low intermittent bleeps. However, unlike the Homer, it cannot be silent when switched on! It will give off its signal continuously but this would enable it to be used as a directional aid in games such as bowls. The sound beacon (catalogue no. 9425) costs £6.38 (concession price).

Perhaps the final word on mobility aids should be that there is no one perfect aid for any blind person to meet all occasions. For example, a guide dog may be perfect for long walks in town and country, but its owner might find it more convenient to go out to a restaurant or to a concert accompanied only with a long cane that can be neatly folded away under a chair. It is obviously not possible to have a guide dog on trial, but the Nottingham Mobility Research Unit is building up a 'library' of hand-held mobility aids which can be borrowed for use under the supervision of a mobility officer. Details from Dr Heyes at the Blind Mobility Research Unit.

Badges
Whether or not it is a good idea for visually handicapped people to wear badges is always a subject for debate. While some blind people hate the idea, others think it does act as a useful symbol to other members of the public, particularly in shops, restaurants, trains or buses and especially for people whose eye defect is not obvious.

Mrs Rosalind Herzfeld, the widow of a blind American judge, designed a badge because of the many occasions on which she and her husband were subjected to embarrassment because people failed to realise that he could not see. Her badge is an oblong shape, two inches long and one inch wide, and shows a hand holding a white stick against a red background. They are available free from the RNIB (which will only take individual orders) or in bulk from *Mrs R.*

Herzfeld, The Penthouse, Flat 4, 21 and 22 Dunraven Street, Park Lane, London W1Y 3FF (tel. 01-493 5367).

The Partially Sighted Society has also produced a badge, showing a partly shaded eye to indicate that the wearer suffers from restricted vision.

Methods of making maps

Blind people finding their way around alone instinctively tend to make use of their other senses to identify landmarks on their route and the kind of information that is valuable to them is not necessarily the same as that which helps a sighted person.

The map that is likely to be most useful is a set of verbal instructions. This can take into account such features as the smell of a fish shop, the gradient of a hill or the sounds associated with a particular location, all difficult to represent on an ordinary map, and warning can be included of such hazards as a protruding hedge. Verbal maps can be recorded on a pocket tape recorder to be played back bit by bit as each stage of the journey is completed.

Maps can also be printed in large type or brailled: an excellent example is the London Underground Guide available from the Royal National Institute for the Blind. It gives lists in braille of the stations on each line as well as other useful information.

Tactile maps and diagrams can be made with a variety of materials, ranging from pieces of string to different grades of sandpaper, and can represent large areas such as whole continents or something as small as the layout of a flat. The RNIB has for a long time provided tactile maps for educational purposes and has more recently begun producing maps of city centres in Britain, starting with London and Birmingham. The value of such maps is in giving a general idea of the shape of an area and the relationship between places.

The possibility of mass-producing maps of particular locations as a mobility aid has been opened up by the advent of the thermoform machine which was designed to make a plastic copy of braille material and can also duplicate tactile maps and diagrams. The idea was developed by the Blind Mobility Research Unit, at the University of Nottingham, and a kit has been compiled for use in conjunction with a thermoform duplicator. Master maps can be made with the kit by a relatively unskilled operator and materials are provided to indicate linear features (roads, paths, railways) point features (traffic lights, bus stops, public lavatories) and area features (park land, pedestrianised street areas, lakes). The kit can also be used for mapping indoor areas such as shopping centres. It costs about £10 and is available from *Dr G. A. James, 223 College Street, Long Eaton, Nottinghamshire NG10 4GF (tel. Long Eaton (060 76) 68974)*.

The Blind Mobility Research Unit has also produced a booklet which gives general information about making various kinds of mobility maps together with instructions on the use of the thermoform kit. It costs £3.50 including postage and is also available from Dr G. A. James (address as above). Duplicating facilities for tactile maps are available at the National Mobility Centre. There is no charge for the use of the thermoform machine: it is only necessary to pay for the cost of the materials.

As these tactile maps take quite a lot of time and effort to produce – but are simple to copy on a thermoform machine – a National Register of Maps for the Visually Handicapped is kept by *Mr A. F. Tatham, The Map Room, Chesham Building, King's College, The Strand, London WC2 2LS*. Anyone wanting to know if a map of a particular area exists should write to Mr Tatham: and all tactile map-makers are asked to register their maps on special forms available from Mr Tatham.

How to guide a blind person
Always let a blind person take a sighted person's arm – not the other way around. Many people, with best intentions, embarrass or even frighten blind people by the way they offer help. It is frightening for a blind person to be grabbed from behind, pushed up steps or frog-marched down them. Also, always ask a blind person if help is wanted. There are a surprising number of well-meaning citizens who will march a blind person across the road without even enquiring first whether he or she wants to go to the other side!

The former Mobility of the Blind Association has produced an excellent illustrated pamphlet showing the correct way to guide a blind person. It starts by explaining that the blind person should always take the sighted person's arm. 'Stand by the side of the blind person with your arms straight, fingers pointing to the ground. Now ask him to take your arm. His hand should grip your arm just above your elbow, so that his fingers are on the inside of your arm and thumb on the outside. His elbow is bent. The grip allows the blind person to be half a pace behind you and he can detect when you are turning, by the movement of your body. There is no need to move your arm.

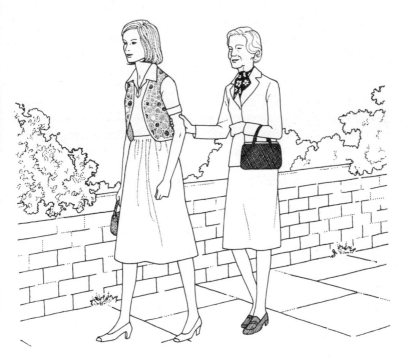

How to guide a blind person
The blind person grips her sighted guide's arm just above the elbow, and walks half a pace behind.

Check that the blind person's toes are pointing in the same direction as yours – if not, you could be parting company!' This is illustrated above.

Doorways
A sighted guide should always approach a door so that the blind person is on the same side as the door hinge; that is, if the hinge is on the left, the blind person should be on the left side of the guide, with the left hand free. The guide goes through the door first and the blind person follows, closing the door with the free hand. The guide opens the door using the hand of the grip arm, and as the handle is turned and the door moves, the blind person can distinguish whether the door is moving inwards or outwards. As the guide starts to walk through, the blind person moves the back of the free (left) hand to the

door, slides it along and contacts the handle, so that after walking through, this hand can be slipped round to the other handle and the door closed.

Stairs

The most common mistake well-meaning people make when guiding a blind person is to say 'steps' without indicating whether they are up or down. The curve of a banister or handrail usually gives warning when the steps are coming to an end. The following technique is recommended for stairs.

To mount a staircase or steps, face the stairs in the normal grip and say 'stairs up'. Step up and place your weight on the first step; as you do so, your partner will feel your arm move slightly upwards – this is the cue to start. As you climb the second step he or she is on the first. Continue walking in rhythm, you being one step in front and your partner's grip arm being slightly stretched forward and upward, until you reach the top . . . then, take a slightly larger stride forward and stop; allowing the blind person to negotiate the last step. As the grip arm resumes its normal position this gives the information you've reached the level again. Going downstairs involves a very similar procedure in which the guide goes ahead one step and the blind person's arm is in a downward tilting position.

Showing a blind person to a seat

Imagine that you are blind: that someone stands you in front of a seat and tells you to sit down – or even worse, pushes you down. You can't see it is safe, and to be pushed down backwards can feel very frightening. A far better way is the following technique suggested for a sighted guide: 'If possible approach the chair centrally, but whether it's from the side, the back or the front, always place your grip hand on the back of the chair. There is no need to tell your partner the position of the back, your arm movement is sufficient. Now, let your partner slide his hand down your arm to the chair back. Your job is now over, it is up to him to move into the chair, feeling the side of it with the calf of the leg and if necessary checking the seat depth with the hand.'

A similar technique is suggested for guiding a blind person into a car. 'There is no need to put your partner into the car; simply place your grip hand on the passenger door handle and tell your partner which way the car is facing. His grip hand then slides down your arm and locates the handle while the other finds the roof. You can now

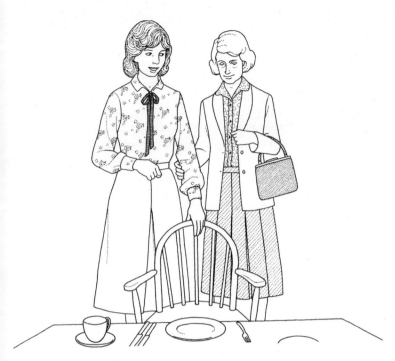

*No need to push a blind person into a seat! Once the guide's hand is on
the back of the chair, a blind person can slide her hand down the guide's
arm to locate the chair, and then move into it unaided.*

walk around to the driving seat. The passenger, having opened the
door and ducked his head, transfers his hand from the roof to the seat,
either steps in, or sits and swings his legs around and finally closes the
door.'

In addition to the examples quoted, the leaflet also explains how to
cope with seating in a restaurant, church or theatre, has hints on
coping with buses and coaches and the best way to approach kerbs as
well as describing the correct way for guide and partner to change
sides.

The pamphlet 'How to Guide a Blind Person' is available from the
RNIB. Another useful publication which gives much more detail
about mobility and guiding techniques is 'See What I Mean', written
by R. B. Foster, a mobility officer in Strathclyde. The booklet costs
30p (but is free to anyone living in the Strathclyde area) and is

obtainable from the *Strathclyde Resource Centre, 276 St Vincent Street, Glasgow G2 5RP (tel. 041-248 5811)*.

Crossing roads
One final piece of advice for the many members of the public who offer to see a blind person across the road. Always cross at safe crossing points and allow plenty of time. Do not leave a blind person standing on the opposite kerb without checking that he or she knows which way they need to go to continue their journey. And, although this may seem obvious, do speak to blind people and identify yourself before taking them across. Policemen and traffic wardens cannot be identified by their voice and often forget that their uniforms mean nothing to a blind person. Do not talk when crossing the road itself; a blind person concentrates on listening to traffic noise and chatter can be distracting. Make it clear when you are leaving. It is rather disconcerting, to say the least, for a blind person to go on talking to the escort who has silently gone away.

★   *If you have a lot of roads to cross, instead of counting, put as many pennies in one of your pockets as you have crossings to make. At each crossing transfer a penny to a pocket on the other side. When you have no pennies left in your original pocket, your journey is completed.*
(Jill Allen, Westcliff-on-Sea)

★   *A spring fastened to a door frame not only prevents the door from being left open so that you bump into it, but it also reduces the fuel bill enough to pay for the door spring.*
(J.F.W. Thomas, Plymouth)

138

Reading

This chapter and the next include all aids to reading and writing for people with limited vision – or with none at all; but the alternatives to reading offered by tape services of various kinds are listed in Chapter 13, *Pleasures of listening* which starts on page 161.

Large print books

It is possible for many people with poor vision to read print if it is larger than normal and clearly printed. The concept of large print books was pioneered nearly twenty years ago by a retired publisher, Mr F. A. Thorpe, who felt he wanted to provide books that would enable people with failing eyesight to continue, or rediscover, the pleasures of reading. The 'Ulverscroft' series of large print books was started in 1964 to provide a range of titles selected from best-selling fiction and non-fiction, in a clear print approximately two and a half times the size of ordinary book print. There are now over thirteen hundred titles in the Ulverscroft series, which is distributed through public libraries but not sold in bookshops – though individuals can buy direct from the publisher, *Ulverscroft Large Print Books, The Green, Bradgate Road, Anstey, Leicester LE7 7FU (tel. Anstey (053-721) 4325)*. Following the success of the Ulverscroft titles, other publishers have begun publishing in large print. They include Cedric Chivers who publish their own large print books, as well as distributing those produced by other British and American publishers. A monthly catalogue is available on request from their *Book Sales Division, 93/100 Locksbrook Road, Bath BA1 3EN (tel. Bath (0225) 316872)*. Other sources of large print books are *George Prior, 37-41 Bedford Row, London WC1R 4JH* and *Magna Print Books, Magna House, Long Preston, North Yorkshire BD23 4ND* from whom catalogues can be obtained on request. A complete list of large print publishers can be requested from the Library Association, which takes an active interest in the provision of material for visually handicapped people. Their free leaflet 'Reading for the Visually Handicapped' provides in large, clear print a guide to the facilities available (send large stamped addressed envelope to *Ann Hobart, Development Secretary, Library Association, 7 Ridgmount Street, London WC1E 7AE*).

The National Library for the Blind also publishes a large print series, named Austin Books, which concentrates on the classics and standard English works. There are about three hundred titles in the Austin series, including history, travel, philosophy and popular science as well as novels. A catalogue is available on request. These books can be borrowed by arrangement through the local public library, not from the Library itself which only lends braille and Moon books direct to readers.

There is also a limited number of reference books available in large print. The Little Oxford Dictionary is available (price £9.25) from Ulverscroft and the Merriam-Webster dictionary, which is published in the United States and therefore has American spellings, is available from George Prior at £15.95. It is estimated that there are now about two thousand large print titles, which is only a minute proportion of the books available to the general population. So although the existence of large print books has effectively reintroduced many visually handicapped readers to their public libraries, there is not nearly enough suitable reading material for those who can only read large print. In a study carried out for the Library Association, it was found that there was not nearly enough non-fiction for the general large print reader nor of books suitable for young readers. It was also pointed out that large print books were too heavy for many elderly people to carry home from a library, and suggested that homes for the elderly, day centres and pensioners' clubs should be encouraged to borrow large print books in bulk for the use of visually handicapped people. Lorna Bell's study 'The Large Print Book and its User', published in 1980 by the Library Association, found that there were many people who were still totally unaware of the existence of large print books – and as these were people who never went into a library, the books must obviously be seen elsewhere in the community if they are to be used by many of the visually handicapped people for whom they were intended.

Libraries vary in the number and variety of large print books they stock. The librarian should be able to help with enquiries about the availability of any particular book in large print. It may also be helpful to know that the Disabled Living Foundation keeps a card-index of large print books and is happy to answer specific queries (e.g. are there any large print cookery books?) though the Foundation does not provide lists of publications. 'Large Type Books in Print' is a comprehensive list of American and many English publications and is published by the *Bowker Publishing Co., PO Box 5, High Street, Epping, Essex CM16 4BU.*

No British newspaper has yet followed the example of the *New York Times*, which publishes a weekly large print edition. There is also a large type edition of the *Readers Digest* magazine available in the United States. In order to obtain these a British reader would need to take out a subscription – payable by international money order. Details from *Large Type Edition, Readers Digest Fund for the Blind Inc., PO Box 241, Mount Morris 61054 Illinois, USA (tel. (815) 734-6963)*. Subscription is $12.95 for 12 months (inc. postage), payable by international money order.

Religious publications

There are a number of large print versions of the complete Bible or individual books. However it is very worthwhile trying to compare all the large print versions available as they vary in type size and thickness of paper. Sometimes it might be better to choose a Bible printed on thicker paper in a less large print as larger print on thin paper may result in confusing shadows from the reverse side. It may also be easier for an elderly person to cope with large print Bibles which are published in individual volumes as these will not be so heavy to handle. Publishers include the *Bible Society, Stonehill Green, Westlea Down, Swindon FN5 7NG (tel. Swindon (0793) 486381)* which has the New Testament in the Authorised Version and in the Good News Bible (Today's English Version) in large print. There is a 40 per cent discount for the blind and partially sighted on direct orders to the Society. A catalogue showing samples of the typefaces used is free on request. *Scripture Gift Mission, Radstock House, Eccleston Street, London SW1W 9LZ (tel. 01-730 2155)* publishes the Gospels and Psalms in exceptionally clear, heavy, black type. Cedric Chivers has published the Gospels and Psalms in large print and the Torch Trust publishes some New Testament books printed in ¼ inch block lettering.

Large print hymn books

The Torch Trust has published a large print edition of *One Hundred Hymns from Christian Praise* (price 40p). Ulverscroft publish a hymn book which is a large print reproduction of the Hospital Hymn Book of the Free Church Federal Council; it contains 119 hymns as well as selected scripture passages and prayers. The book is similar in size to an ordinary hymn book and contains an index which offers cross-references to six of the most generally used hymn books. The *Ulvers-*

croft Large Print Hymn Book costs £1.50. The *Ulverscroft Large Print Song Book* also contains a small selection of hymns and carols in addition to many popular old time songs (price 95p). Cedric Chivers has a large print edition of the Methodist Hymn Book (price £6.25).

Braille

This system of embossed script, which has been universally adopted by blind people, was invented by a Frenchman, Louis Braille, in 1824. It consists, in its English version, of sixty-three symbols which are variations on the dots of a domino six. Apart from the twenty-six letters of the alphabet, the symbols include eight braille punctuation signs and twenty-seven contractions for such common combinations of letters as 'st' or 'th'. There are two grades – Grade One, in which every word is fully spelt, and Grade Two, the everyday form in which various contractions are used to express frequently recurring groups of letters and words and thus reduce the bulk of the braille.

To read braille by touch, a person has to develop a sensitivity in the fingertips which may not always come easily. It has been estimated that only a small proportion (about 20 per cent) of the blind population can read it but, given determination, age is no barrier. It might be worth noting that when an 84-year-old clergyman wrote to *In Touch* that he was making very slow progress in learning to read braille and wondered whether other listeners had managed it at his age, the *In Touch* office was inundated with letters from blind listeners in all parts of the country who assured him that they had learnt braille when in their seventies and eighties and found they derived a great deal of pleasure from it. Even if braille reading is too slow for the enjoyment of books, it can be useful for other pursuits, such as playing cards (see Chapter 14, page 181) or making labels.

Help in learning braille

There are several possible sources of help in learning to read and write braille. First, it is worth enquiring whether the local social services have a braille specialist available. Since the 1971 reorganisation of the social services many areas are expecting their 'blind welfare specialists' to cope also with the wide variety of work that comes into the social services departments. As a result very few social workers have been able to give time to individual braille tuition as the home teachers used to do. But in some areas, the local authority organises braille classes at day or rehabilitation centres. Elsewhere the local evening institutes may run classes in braille and as with other subjects if classes do not exist and there is sufficient demand (usually about twelve students) the local education authority is obliged to provide it.

There are also a number of 'do-it-yourself' possibilities. David Scott Blackhall, the first compere of *In Touch*, managed to teach himself braille with the aid of a manual produced by the RNIB. This book, *How To Learn to Read*, is available on request from the RNIB. It introduces braille in either 'giant character' dots (catalogue no. 12) or intermediate size dots (catalogue no. 3798) and has inkprint explanations.

A course of taped lessons on 'beginning braille' has been devised by Dr Michael Tobin of the Centre for the Education of the Visually Handicapped. The course consists of twenty lessons recorded on to two cassettes, with a book of twenty sheets of braille, corresponding to the lessons. The course is free. Anyone who owns a cassette recorder and wishes to learn braille by this method should send two C90 cassettes, or the equivalent in cash, to the producer, *Torchlight, BBC Radio Manchester, PO Box 90, Oxford Road, Manchester M60 1SJ*. He will copy the lessons on to the cassettes and supply the braille booklet. For those who have a talking book machine, *Beginning Braille* is also available as a talking book and can be obtained on request (catalogue no. 2915) from the British Talking Book Service. Suggestions for useful follow-up material, as well as alternative 'teach yourself' books are contained in a leaflet, 'Beginning Braille', obtainable from the RNIB Students Library. The Centre for the Education of the Visually Handicapped in Birmingham, directed by Dr Michael Tobin, takes a particular interest in braille teaching methods. While most of its work is concerned with the teaching of children, some of the methods being tried in schools might well be of interest to adults or those teaching them.

Braille publishers
There are a great many braille publications – both books and magazines. The biggest publishers are the RNIB (which has the advantage of a computer to do some of the work), the National Library for the Blind, and the Scottish Braille Press. Between 500 and 800 titles are published in braille each year, but probably the most widely read braille publication is the braille *Radio Times*, which is sent free each week to about 5,000 people.

Braille publications

The RNIB's publications cover a wide field from children's books and dictionaries to language textbooks, vocational handbooks for cane-workers or gardeners to specialist publications on the law, medicine and philosophy. Complete catalogues are available on request, but perhaps the most important point for braille readers to note is that all proposed publications are announced in two RNIB journals: the braille *Monthly Announcements* or the print *New Beacon*, and it is only if sufficient orders are placed that the books are published.

The Scottish Braille Press is responsible for a wide variety of publications. It publishes six braille periodicals, including three weeklies, and in addition prints and distributes another three dozen magazines on behalf of various organisations concerned with the welfare of the blind. It also has its own 'Thistle' paperback series which produces a popular novel each month. Its range of book publications is growing steadily and includes books of knitting patterns and cookery recipes which are very much in demand. The Press has always practised positive discrimination in employing either blind or disabled workers. In 1981 all but six of its fifty-nine employees were either blind or disabled. All workers are paid in accordance with printing trade wage agreements and the conditions under which the staff work, both as regards premises and equipment, compare favourably with any modern factory.

The National Library for the Blind is the main source of books for braille readers. Its 350,000 volumes are available free to all blind readers. The library issues full catalogues and the Braille Library Bulletin which comes out six times a year (annual subscription 25p) gives up-to-date information on all new additions.

Quite a number of local voluntary associations keep small stocks of braille books, available on loan, which might be particularly helpful to beginners. The Torch Trust for the Blind has a library of evangelical literature.

The RNIB Students' Braille Library

This is a library of braille books, which is primarily intended to provide study material for blind students at universities or other places of further education, including part-time evening classes, and also to meet the needs of professional workers. Books from the Students' Braille Library can also be borrowed by any other blind person: though priority in borrowing is always given to a student.

Quite a number of textbooks in common use, as well as a variety of books of academic interest, are available. The library contains over 57,000 braille volumes in a number of languages, and the catalogue is currently undergoing revision; but the sections on biography, history, social sciences, English and foreign languages are already available.

Other material needed for studies can also be transcribed on request, though obviously it is advisable to give as much notice as possible to ensure that books are received on time as it can take several months to transcribe a book into braille. Transcriptions are done by volunteer braillists and people interested in doing this work should contact the Braille Transcription Manager, Elizabeth Twining, for details of training. It can take up to a year to train someone to be proficient as a braille transcriber, so only those really prepared to devote a lot of time and effort should apply. A knowledge of foreign languages or a mathematical or scientific background is particularly valuable.

Transcription services
One group of voluntary braillists who do work for the Students' Library are also available for help with transcribing letters to and from blind people and their relatives and friends. They can also handle books and magazine articles of all kinds and even knitting patterns or chess. They can braille in modified codes in several languages including French, German, Spanish, and Latin. There is a minimal charge for paper and overheads and a charge is made for duplicating. Full details can be obtained from the *Voluntary Transcribers Group, c/o A. C. Hackshaw, 4 Shreenwater Cottages, Old Hollow, Mere, Wiltshire (tel. Mere (0747) 860573)*.

There are two other services run by volunteers who will transcribe into braille, books or other material for blind people: *The Leeds Braille Group (Secretary Mrs Lilian Bennett), 15 Fearnville Close, Leeds, West Yorkshire LS8 3HG (tel. Leeds (0532) 657350)* and the *Yorkshire Braille Service (Secretary Mrs B. Jackson), 49 Sandhill Oval, Leeds LS17 8EF (tel. Leeds (0532) 684863)*. The *Prison Braille Unit Service* which operates at Wakefield Prison for the north of the country and at Aylesbury Prison for the south is also willing to undertake work and charge only for the cost of the materials. Enquiries to the *Education Officer, H.M. Prison* either at *Love Lane, Wakefield, West Yorkshire* or at *Bierton Road, Aylesbury, Buckinghamshire*.

Urgently needed material of a non-technical nature can be transcribed by the RNIB's Short Document Service. However this service is limited to one document of not more than 3,000 words per person per month – though up to ten copies of any document will be sent. Other material may be accepted when the capacity of the service permits. Enquiries to *RNIB Short Document Service, Braille House, 338-46 Goswell Road, London EC1V 7JE*.

Moon

The other embossed system of reading, which many older people find easier to learn, is Moon. This system, invented in 1847 by the blind Dr William Moon, consists of large simplified Roman letters. It is a clear, bold type but, unlike braille, it cannot be written by the ordinary person so it is not as perfect a communication method. Moon is slower to produce than braille and far less literature is available. The main printer of Moon material is the Moon Branch of the RNIB at *Holmesdale Road, Reigate, Surrey RH2 0BA*, which will supply a full catalogue of books on request. Moon books can be borrowed from the National Library for the Blind.

The Moon Branch also produces a number of weekly and monthly publications including *Moon Newspaper*, a weekly summary of the news, specially designed for deaf-blind readers; *Diane*, a women's magazine; *Moon Messenger*, a religious publication; and two monthlies, *The Moon Magazine* and *The Light of the Moon*, which both reproduce articles from national newspapers. All Moon books and periodicals are free.

As Moon cannot be written by hand, the Moon branch offers to transcribe private letters of not more than 600 words at the rate of 15p per 150 words. It is also possible to arrange for birthday, Christmas or other greetings cards to be embossed in Moon.

Learning Moon
The local authority social services department is supposed to provide Moon teaching, as well as braille teaching, as part of their rehabilitation service for blind people. But for people living in areas where specialist help is non-existent, the Moon branch issues a free do-it-yourself packet called *The Moon System* by Hilda Bradfield, with an inkprint booklet of tips for learners. Many older people have found it quite easy to learn Moon. Like braille, Moon comes in two grades: Grade One is mainly uncontracted and a selection of short stories,

knitting patterns, devotional literature and even some full-length novels are available. Grade Two Moon has forty-five contractions, but these are not difficult to learn and are often a matter of common sense. A much wider range of books and magazines is available in Grade Two Moon. Even if people do not want to read books in Moon, a knowledge of the alphabet will enable them to use Moon playing cards.

Reading machines

The arrival of the new technology, made possible by the micro-chip, has led to a number of exciting developments in reading and writing equipment for the blind. The new writing equipment (described more fully on pages 156–7) can be used only by people who are familiar with braille, but at least one of the reading machines has brought new opportunities for people who cannot read braille.

The Kurzweil

The first talking/reading machine, the Kurzweil, was invented by an American team led by Raymond Kurzweil in 1974.

The Kurzweil reading machine (KRM) has a miniature electronic camera which transmits the images from the printed page to a small computer built into the machine, which converts it into synthetic speech. The machine can 'read' up to 250 words a minute, or be slowed down to spell out words if required. But it is not yet the miracle machine that will translate any and every page of print to give a blind person complete access to all books. Research carried out in Britain during 1979/80 showed the machine's limitations as well as its achievements. A Kurzweil reading machine was given a year's trial in a research project jointly sponsored by the RNIB and St Dunstan's in which 200 blind people of all ages had the opportunity to try the machine. The final report pointed out that the Kurzweil machine could only read clear, dark print on a light background. It could not read handwritten or typewritten material or newsprint, nor could it cope well with italic print. But given suitable material the various blind people who tried it found that after they had got used to the synthetic voice, they could 'read' easily and at a reasonable speed. A number of children took part in the trials, but there was a dearth of suitable material for them. The Kurzweil cannot cope with pictures so that many children's books, where the print is broken up by illustrations, are not suitable for reading on the machine.

The report's final assessment was that the most likely use for the Kurzweil machine would be as a resource in a school, college or library where it could be made available to a number of users. At its price of £17,000 it is not likely to be bought by many private individuals, but it could be a valuable tool to blind professional and office workers if it were available at their place of work. One blind man who assessed it pointed out that it would be particularly valuable for a blind person who did not have a secretary or other sighted assistant. Further information about the Kurzweil can be obtained from St Dunstan's or the RNIB or from the British agents, *Omnifont International Ltd, 12 High Street, Chalfont St Giles (tel. 02407 5995)*.

The Optacon

The reading machine which has had more world-wide use is the Optacon, which was invented in 1970 by an American electronics engineer, Professor John Linville, to help his blind daughter. The Optacon is designed to convert the image of a printed letter into a tactile form that a blind person can feel with one finger. The Optacon (a name derived from OPtical TActile CONverter) has three main sections, a miniature opto-electric camera, an electronics section and a tactile, stimulator array. The machine is about the size of a large book and weighs four pounds. In order to 'read', the camera – which is only about the size of a pocket knife – is held in the user's right hand and moved slowly across the line of print, while the fingers of the left hand are put over the main part of the machine which houses the electronics. The tactile stimulator array has tiny metal rods which can all vibrate independently, and the tips of the rods protrude through holes in the machine's plastic cover, so grooved that one finger can touch the entire array. When the machine is working, the image of the printed letter is converted into a pattern of vibrating rods, felt on the tip of the user's forefinger.

The obvious value of the Optacon is that it gives independent access to the printed word for a blind person, but learning to read with an Optacon requires a period of training followed by intensive practice. It is not a fast method of reading. There were about 300 Optacons in use in Britain in 1981, and it was estimated that the speed with which people read using this varied between ten and eighty words a minute; but the average person could not read much faster than twenty or thirty words a minute. To read with the Optacon demands a very sensitive touch, so although its output relates to print and not braille, the sensitivity required to 'read' the vibrating rods is as great as – if not greater – than that needed to read braille. While one does not need to know braille to read with an Optacon, it is not the solution for those who have not managed to read by other tactile methods. But even slow reading with an Optacon may well be preferable to having to wait for someone else to help, particularly when a blind person needs to refer to short items in print. Quite a number of computer programmers are using Optacons at work, as the Optacon also has an attachment with which a Visual Display Unit display can be read. It is also possible to get a lens module to attach to a typewriter to enable a blind person to fill out printed forms or correct typescript, and a magnifier module to help with the reading of extremely small print.

The basic Optacon costs about £2,200 (plus VAT) and training programmes are available for people who need it for work or study purposes either through the RNIB's Commercial Training College, or through Electronic Aids for the Blind, an independent charity set up in 1978 to help provide Optacons, and other electronic aids, for blind children and adults, and to instruct them in their use. A number of schools for the blind are now giving Optacon training to some of their pupils, but on the whole British schools still regard Optacon reading as an extra skill, often taught out of school hours. By contrast, on the Continent – particularly in Italy and West Germany – and in the United States, blind children are given intensive training with Optacon machines from an early age and Optacons are part of the equipment used to help blind children attend ordinary schools. In Italy where a research project monitored the progress of several hundred Optacon students, it was reported that after continuous use of between six months to one year, the average reading speed achieved was forty-four words a minute, compared to only thirteen to nineteen words a minute after the initial training had been completed. Brian Payne, a British computer programmer/analyst, who started Electronic Aids for the Blind after he had visited the United States on a Winston Churchill Fellowship feels passionately that the key to integration of blind people in ordinary schools and a wider range of jobs, lies in the increasing use of equipment such as the Optacon. For more details about the work done by the EAB write to *Brian Payne, 28 Crofton Avenue, Orpington, Kent BR6 8DU* (tel. (evenings and weekends only) Farnborough (0689) 55651). The Optacon is made by Telesensory Systems Inc. of California. The British agent is *John Tillisch, 10 Barleymow Passage, London W4 (tel. 01-994 6477).* In

1981, TSI in the United States was assessing some prototype speech synthesiser units which could be attached to an Optacon and would obviously greatly enhance its value. But it is not yet known when this talking Optacon unit is likely to be available.

★   *As labels large enough for a partially-sighted gardener to read would look rather unsightly in flowerbeds, use strips of insulating tape instead. It is available in various bright colours as well as black and white, from electrical suppliers, and the different coloured strips can be used to indicate different species.*
(Miss M.C. Thornton, Bishopsteignton, Devon)

★   *To mark your place in a braille book, fasten a paper clip alongside the appropriate line.*
(David Scott Blackhall)

★   *The big plastic laundry bags make ideal carriers for heavy braille books.*
(Peter White)

Aids to writing

This chapter looks at ways in which people can write, and make identifying marks or labels. It is not always appreciated that even a minimal knowledge of braille can be useful for purposes of labelling and many people retain sufficient vision to be able to write, if they choose a suitable method.

Felt pens: The use of these, rather than of ordinary ink pens or ballpoints, may make it easier for someone who can still see a limited amount to read what he or she has written. As people with limited sight often have to write with the eyes (and nose) close to the paper, it is worth looking out for the felt pens which are water- rather than spirit-based. An advisory service on the best type of pen to use for different types of work is offered by one manufacturer, who states that he would also be happy to advise visually handicapped people on their special needs. Contact John Storrs, *Berol Ltd*, Oldmedow Rd, *Kings Lynn* PE30 4JR (tel. Kings Lynn (0553) 61221).

Writing frames: These, and *raised line paper*, both produced by the RNIB, can help solve the problem of writing in a straight line.

Lined writing paper: A paper with *very* dark lines can be bought from the Partially Sighted Society; and also from F.C. Mills Ltd, who are prepared to deal with individual customers but prefer to deal with bulk orders from organisations or groups. The paper is packed in reams (500 sheets), and the firm cannot supply less than one ream at a time. The price for a ream of A4 paper is £3.70 (plus VAT). Address: *F.C. Mills Ltd, P.O. Box 17, Wetherby, West Yorkshire LS23 7BY (tel. Boston Spa (0937) 63140)*.

Typing
Those who have learnt to touch type before their sight began to fail will have no difficulty in operating the machine, but may find it difficult to read what they have written.

Heavily-inked typewriter ribbons: These make type-written letters clearer. All typewriter ribbons are made in three settings – light,

151

medium and heavy – but the last is not always available. In case of difficulty, they can be ordered by post (specify make and model of typewriter) from *MAMBA (Midlands) Ltd, Millfields House, Lichfield Road, Tamworth, Staffordshire B79 7SR (tel. Tamworth (0827) 60931).*

Enlargement: Visually handicapped typists may find it helpful to use aids which either enlarge the material from which they are copying, or which magnify their own typescript. It is possible to get a variety of copyholders which incorporate a magnifying reading bar from *Data Presentation Co., 49-51 Brewhouse Hill, Wheathampstead, Hertford-shire AL4 8AN (tel. Wheathampstead (058 283) 2471).*

There are several industrial magnifiers which can be fitted over typewriters so that typists can see their work enlarged, but these are rather bulky and because of their size do not give very powerful magnification.

A copyholder (which does not magnify) stocked by most office suppliers can be very useful for holding the copy up close to the eyes: the Myers Copyholder, for instance, costs £12.50 (including VAT) from Rymans, who will offer a discount on bulk orders.

The Disabled Living Foundation's information service should be able to provide details of models and manufacturers of copy-holders.

Large print typewriters: There is a number of large print typewriters, all rather expensive, but they might be worth considering if their use would mean that a person with low vision could read what had been written. It is obviously important to look carefully at the various type-faces available to see which is really best for a particular person's use. Among the large print typewriters available is the Brother electric model 5513, which is available to partially sighted people at a special discount price of £315 (normal price £450). This machine is fitted with Bulletin type, which gives six letters to the inch. There is also a special keyboard shield available which ensures that individual keys only are depressed, so that each key can be selected without touching an adjacent one. This shield, which costs £29, is also of great use to those who are without full control of their fingers. Enquiries to *Bennett Typewriter Company, 27 Lewisham Way, New Cross, London SE14 (tel. 01-692 4941).*

IBM make a Selectric (golf-ball) typewriter with Orator type, which gives ten letters to the inch. The type-face on this machine yields capital letters one-fifth of an inch high. It costs £508 (plus VAT). Full details from *IBM Ltd, 101 Wigmore Street, London W17H 0AB (tel. 01-935 6600)*.

Olivetti produce a manual typewriter fitted with a jumbo type-face giving eight letters to the inch, and with an extra long (fifteen-inch) carriage. This machine, the Linea 98, costs £439, but there is a considerable discount for people buying through a social services department or local education authority. Details from *British Olivetti, Government and National Accounts Department, 17-29 Sun Street, London EC2M 2PU (tel. 01-377 8644)*.

Another manual portable typewriter is the Mini-Jumbo Easy Typer, which has been specially designed as a large print typewriter for use in schools. It produces very clear letters and numerals – ten letters to the inch – and costs £107.25 (plus VAT). Details from *OEM (Reprographic), 133/49 St Nicholas Circle, Leicester LE1 4LE (tel. 0533 50481)*.

As there are frequent changes in the style of large type-faces and the machines available, it might be worth checking for up-to-date details with the information service of the Disabled Living Foundation in London.

It is possible to buy a limited range of typewriters at a discount through the RNIB, and details can be obtained through the sales manager. But it is probably cheaper to get equipment from an ordinary discount store. The RNIB does not undertake any after-sales service.

People unable to afford a typewriter may find the local voluntary society willing to help with a grant, or the loan of a machine. A student might get help from either the local education department, or from one of the educational charities (see Chapter 17, *Education*). The Manpower Services Commission has funds available in certain circumstances (see Chapter 3, *Employment*).

Typing, like braille, is taught to newly-blind people in the home, in some areas, or at a local rehabilitation centre. But if this is not available it should not be too difficult to find local evening classes. As typing is taught to people with normal sight by touch methods a blind student may well be able to follow the class. However, unlike classes at rehabilitation centres, which usually arrange transport for their students, the evening classes would expect blind students to make their own travel arrangements. (See page 154 for braille aids to typing.)

For braille readers, Pitman's *Teach Yourself Typing* is available from the RNIB, who also supply free a plastic chart showing the layout of a standard keyboard. The RNIB can supply braille scales to order for most makes of typewriter, and stocks a selected range of adapted typewriters at special rates for blind people. These are fitted with braille scales (useful for margin setting and tabulation), and metal studs to mark the home keys – a great help for beginners. Incidentally, a lot of blind typists find it quite easy to locate the home keys when they are marked with pieces of sticking plaster.

A typing course on tape is available from the Tape Recording Service for the Blind (see page 171–2).

Braille writing machines
Braillists can get their basic writing equipment from the RNIB. This ranges from hand frames, small enough to be carried in the pocket, to more elaborate machines almost equivalent in size and weight to a typewriter.

Hand frames: The operator has to make each individual dot with a stylus or 'dotter' from the opposite side of the paper by indenting them – thus the characters have to be written the wrong way round from right to left. So one starts using a hand frame by learning to write braille in reverse – it surprises most people that this comes quite naturally after a while! But it takes a much longer time and a lot of practice to acquire a reasonable speed. The RNIB produces a number of writing frames ranging in price (to blind persons) from £3.04 to 22p.

Faced with the problem of learning to write in a totally different way, a newly blind person may well feel that the task is insuperable; and for the older man or woman past working age it is often considered that the effort of learning to write braille is only worth while if it is needed to maintain a job. But in fact there are many ways in which the ability to write even a few words of braille may make a lot of difference: in making a note of an address or telephone number – and perhaps above all for labelling (see page 81).

Stainsby: The pocket frames have the advantage of being easily carried about, but the braille writing machines are rather heavy. All standard braille machines have six keys which represent the six dots of the braille cell, and the first three fingers of each hand are used for operating the six keys. The machine which has for many years been regarded as the standard piece of braille writing equipment is the British-made Stainsby. It is an easy machine to use. Braille is written exactly as it is read, and although the dots are punched down into the page and therefore written from right to left, it is not necessary to write backwards as with the hand frames. The only major disadvantage of the machine, in the opinion of many users, is that it is too noisy.

There are Stainsby machines for writing both interpoint and interline braille and this may be the appropriate place to explain the difference between them. In the case of interpoint, the lines of braille are little more than half a cell apart and the braille on the reverse side of the page is embossed with the dots between the dots of the front page. For beginners, this is not quite so easy to read as interline braille, where the lines of braille are more than the height of a braille cell apart and the braille on the reverse side of the sheet is embossed between the lines of the braille on the first page.

Unfortunately at the time of writing most types of Stainsby machines were unavailable as the RNIB had not been able to find a firm willing to undertake the manufacture of the Stainsby machines though the Institute is continuing its search.

Perkins: This is an alternative machine, imported by the RNIB from the United States, and very much more expensive. In July 1981, the standard model of Perkins brailler cost £63.88 (or £75.36 with its carrying case) whereas the Stainsby machines available (both inter-pointing models) cost only £19.28 or £21.47.

However, while it is more expensive, the Perkins is a much more sophisticated machine than the Stainsby. To begin with, it has the considerable advantage of being an upward writer, so that the braille can be read while the paper is in the machine. Its operation is rather different from the Stainsby, but not very difficult to learn. Unlike the Stainsby, it has a back-space key, a line spacer and a carriage return lever, all situated at the front of the machine. It is also much less noisy than the Stainsby models. It produces braille spaced as for interpointing, but using one side of the paper only. It is also possible to get a 'Jumbo' Perkins, price £86.64, which produces the extra-large braille which is particularly helpful for beginners.

Marburg: A new upward braille writer which the RNIB were planning in 1981 to import from West Germany. This machine, which looks rather more attractive than other braille writers, is also more versatile. It is possible to braille directly on to postcards or Dymo tape, and the Marburg writer has a margin guide which enables the user to space work out accurately without counting, as one would have to on a Perkins or Stainsby. The Marburg writer does however require a heavier striking action than the other braille writers, so that some people, particularly children, may not find it so easy to use. It is lighter than a Perkins, and fits neatly into a flat carrying case. The cost of the Marburg writer will be about £40.

Temory: There is one piece of braille writing equipment which to some extent bridges the gap between the writing machines and the hand frames. Neither of these are really ideally suited for students or others who need to take notes and also move about a lot in the course of their work. A Japanese writing frame, the Temory, which the RNIB first imported in 1981, is light and easy to carry, and has its own supply of paper dispensed from a roll on the left of the brailling surface. Once brailling is completed, the paper can be cut off against the frame's serrated edge and stored on a hook on one side of the frame. Another constant problem of hand frame users is the ease with which the stylus is lost – the Temory frame is partly magnetised, so that its stylus should stay put! The Temory frame costs £1.92 (catalogue no. 9018).

Paperless braille

One of the major disadvantages of braille is its bulk. Not only are most of the writing machines cumbersome, but the braille book takes up much more space than its print equivalent. A braille version of the Little Oxford Dictionary comes to sixteen hefty volumes, and the Bible consists of seventy-two braille books which would occupy nine foot of shelving. It was therefore a tremendous breakthrough when a French couple, Oleg and Andrée Tretiakoff, who were working on a computer-assisted method for transcribing French literature into braille, realised that paper was not necessary for people to read braille: what was needed was to have a series of raised dots appropriately positioned, and capable of being moved up and down to show the presence or absence of a dot.

Digicassette: A development of the Tretiakoffs' first portable braille recorder. It is about the same size as an ordinary cassette recorder, but it has a tactile reading bar on which braille is displayed on a line with twenty braille characters. The braille is stored on a cassette (the kind used for hi-fi recordings) and written into the machine using the seven bar keyboard (one for each braille dot and a space bar) which is built into the front of the machine. The braille is presented in the tactile bar as it is written and it can then be transferred, either manually or automatically, to the cassette. The storage capacity is immense – using a C90 cassette, the Digicassette will hold the equivalent of 1,000 pages of braille. The information stored on the cassette can be easily located for recall on the tactile bar as the machine incorporates an indexing system.

At the time or writing, there was a six-month delay in getting the machines over to Britain, and no model was available in this country for examination. But the British agents are hopeful that it will be possible to import the machines in the not too distant future. Full details from *Erleybridge Communications Ltd, 3rd Floor, 2-4 Old Street, London EC1V 9AA (tel. 01-250 1928).*

Versabraille: Another similar machine now available in Britain is the American designed Versabraille. This records and stores braille in similar fashion to the Digicassette. It has capacity for indexing the braille material so that the right line of braille can be accurately recalled. This means, for example, that a blind office worker can use a machine like this for keeping a diary, or detailed lists, catalogues or directories which can be referred to literally at the touch of a switch. The Versabraille can also be used like a word processor to edit and correct material without the necessity of re-writing entire texts, and with extra attachments can convert braille into print or vice versa. The Versabraille also has an audio capacity – so that material can be recorded on to the tape, with braille indexing for easy retrieval. The basic equipment costs about £4,000 and in 1981 fewer than a dozen people in Britain had their own machine. But in France about three hundred Digicassettes were in use, and a German machine, the Braillex, not yet available in Britain, was being quite widely used in West German schools. Full details of Versabraille from *Telesensory Systems (Inc.), 10 Barleymow Passage, London W4 (tel. 01-994 6467).*

Brailink: In addition to these portable systems – which can be used by people who have no access to a computer – there are bigger and more expensive systems designed to be used by computer programmers.

Clarke & Smith (who make the talking book machines) have produced Brailink which has a standard typewriter keyboard so that it can be used by people with no knowledge of braille. Full details from *Clarke & Smith, Melbourne Road, Wallington, Surrey SM6 85D (tel. 01-669 4411)*.

BITS. Another system in which braille and inkprint can be produced simultaneously has been devised by Dr John Gill of the Warwick Research Unit for the Blind. The braille it produces is not quite the same as Grade 2, but is claimed to be a good approximation. Full information about BITS (braille and ink-print text processing system) can be obtained from Erleybridge Communications (see *Digicassette*, page 157, for address).

Talking aids: It is the possibility of translating braille into print – and vice versa – as well as the speed with which braille reference material can be retrieved from cassette storage that opens up a whole new range of educational and career opportunities for blind children and adults, if someone is able and willing to pay the rather high price of the equipment. The other advance in technology affecting blind people is the possibility of speech output on a variety of equipment. In 1976, Telesensory Systems produced the Speech-plus calculator and in 1981 a Japanese-made talking calculator, which costs £85, also appeared on the British market. Details from *Panasonic Business Equipment, 107-109 Whitby Road, Slough, Berkshire (tel. Slough (0753) 75841)*. Other talking aids available include the IBM talking typewriter. This is really an audio unit that can be attached to their word processing equipment. The talking typewriter will read back, either in letters or in words, whatever has been typed and so allows blind typists to review and correct their own work. Once again this is expensive equipment – the audio unit costs £2,814.

Because these systems are new and rapidly changing it is difficult to assess their full implications, but both the British Computer Association for the Blind and Electronic Aids for the Blind are likely to be well informed about new equipment as it becomes available, and anyone interested in finding out more details would be well advised to contact them for up-to-date guidance.

Another source of advice is the Technical Department of the RNIB, which has appointed an electronics engineer to advise on systems suitable for the blind.

Correspondence clubs

There are several braille correspondence clubs. Roy Tweed has been running one since 1947 and states that he has 700 members aged between twenty and eighty from all walks of life, at home and abroad. Details from him at *51 Brynifor Estate, Mountain Ash, Glamorgan (tel. Mountain Ash (0443) 472939)*.

In 1976 a Newcastle social worker started a similar club to give new braillists an opportunity to use their skills. Anyone interested should write to *Mrs Linda Watts, Social Services Department, Civic Centre, Barras Bridge, Newcastle upon Tyne NE99 2BM (tel. Newcastle (0632) 328520, ext. 6320/6321)*.

Other alphabets

Moon

The other well known embossed alphabet, Moon, cannot be written by an individual, though the Moon Society will undertake to emboss individual private letters (see page 146).

Fishburne alphabet

A few years ago an American engineer, Sam Fishburne, invented a very simple alphabet which can be written on a special embossing machine. The Fishburne alphabet was devised for use by blind people who do not know braille, and who would like a simple way of labelling or making short notes. It is not suitable for longer texts. The symbols consist of dots, vertical lines, horizontal lines and diagonal lines. The alphabet is divided into groups of six letters. A is a dot above the line, B a dot below the line, C a dot above and below the line. D, E and F are two dots above, below, and above and below the line. The next six letters of the alphabet are shown similarly with vertical lines, followed by horizontal and diagonal lines in the same manner. There are special symbols for Y and Z. The symbols are quite large and designed to be easily felt. Details of the alphabet, and a cassette explaining the system, as well as the special embosser, can be ordered via the RNIB's sales department (though it is not a stock item in its catalogue of aids and equipment). More details about the alphabet can be obtained from the inventor's son, *C.C. Fishburne, 221 North Gordon Drive, Winston Salem, North Carolina, 27104, USA (tel. (919) 765 2938)*.

Labelling devices

In addition to the embossed alphabets, there are a variety of ways in which visually handicapped people can read short messages, or labels. Large print labels can be made with an industrial Dymo machine – the Esselte Dymo 2300 signmaker. The letters are ½ inch high on ¾ inch tape, and as well as being large and clear enough to be read by some people with residual vision, others with a very sensitive touch may even be able to read them by feel. The labeller is too expensive for individuals to buy for their own exclusive use (it costs about £159 plus VAT) but it might be worth considering by a club or other institution used by a lot of visually handicapped people. Garages and other workshops often own these signmakers and might be willing to make labels for a partially sighted person on request. Self adhesive raised letters which can be used to mark items or to spell out short messages can be bought in stationers, and good toyshops may have magnetic letters which can be used on metal surfaces. One could improvise a simple message 'pad' with such letters on a metal tray – or 'write' an essential telephone number down in brightly coloured numerals on the door of a refrigerater.

A recent American invention which has a lot of potential for labelling and 'tactile' writing and drawing is Hi-marks, a bright orange fluorescent substance which is dispensed in a small tube with a fine nozzle. It can be squeezed out of the tube to make signs, symbols, or to draw lines as required. It will adhere to a variety of surfaces including metal, plastic, paper or fabric, and will harden within 2/3 hours after application so that one is left with a permanently attached, raised, vividly coloured mark or drawing. It can only be applied easily by a sighted person, but the very bright colour combined with the raised line or mark make it easy for blind or partially sighted people to appreciate. Hi-marks is made by the *Mark-Tex Corporation, 161 Coolidge Avenue, Englewood, New Jersey 07631, USA*, and is available in Britain from the Partially Sighted Society.

A large variety of labelling methods is available to braillists. The RNIB sells different types of labelling materials, and most of them are easy to use in conjunction with the single line guide (catalogue no. 9027). Jessica Finch, a blind teacher, has made a special study of labelling methods suitable for blind people, both braillists and non-braillists. She has designed a portable exhibition to demonstrate her ideas, and the equipment that is available. More details from *Mrs Finch, 24 Norwich Street, Cambridge (tel. 0223 51910).*

Pleasures of listening

The spoken word, whether recorded on tape or received via radio or television, is the main source of information and entertainment for visually handicapped people unable to read print. This chapter lists some of the sources from which one can get equipment or recordings available to the blind. In recent years there has been a tremendous increase in the amount of recorded material, but unfortunately it is not always easy to know what is available as there is as yet no central register of spoken word recordings. In an attempt to overcome this problem, the Talking Newspaper Association in 1981 appointed an Information Officer to compile a central register of tape services and once this is established it should provide a comprehensive guide of specialist material available to the blind.

Broadcasting

Radio
This is obviously the perfect medium for blind people, and all registered blind people are eligible for a radio set on free permanent loan, under the terms of the British Wireless for the Blind Fund. The Fund does not issue radio sets to partially sighted people. There are two sets currently available: one is a mains radio (the RM33) which has preselected press button tuning and the other set issued by the Fund is a portable, battery operated radio (the RT22). Both sets have long, medium and VHF wavebands. In addition a small personal transistor set is available for blind people who are bed-ridden or confined to a wheel-chair, and who would find the ordinary sets too heavy or bulky to handle.

The Wireless for the Blind Fund is prepared through its local agents to issue four free PP9 batteries a year to any blind person who has one of the Fund's radio sets. In addition, the local agency – which is usually either the local voluntary organisation for the blind or the local social services department – can buy from the Fund further supplies of batteries at concession prices. As this agreement is left to the discretion of the local agency, the availability of cheap batteries varies considerably around the country.

The Fund also provides stethophones (ear phones) free to those blind people who could not listen to their radio without disturbing other people and to those who have slight hearing loss. The stethophones do not amplify the sound output and would not help people whose hearing loss is severe enough to necessitate the use of hearing aids.

Aids to enable people with a severe hearing loss to listen to the radio include adaptors in the form of light-weight stethophones or hearing aids which are wired into the radio. These give users their own volume control and can also have a transformer cutting out the volume altogether so that others cannot hear the radio at all. These adaptations must be installed by an electrician. Another aid has the advantage of allowing the user freedom of movement within the room in which he or she is listening. This loop system involves running a wire around the perimeter of the room with a transformer attached to a mains radio, television, talking book machine or tape recorder. The output is heard directly through the user's hearing aid without affecting other people in the room. The Medresco behind-the-ear hearing aid is particularly suited to this system, but the adaptations must again be installed by an expert.

There is also an aid which can be installed without technical expertise. This is a microphone aid, and consists of stethophones connected to a small amplifier with a volume control and connected in turn by a long lead to a miniature microphone which sticks on the loudspeaker grille of a radio or television set. This equipment cost about £30 in 1981. The component parts needed for the other adaptations are not so expensive, but there would be an installation charge. Members of the Talking Book Library would be able to call on the volunteer engineer to install a loop system for their talking book machines, and he might be willing to adapt the system for a radio or television set too.

Details of these aids are given in a booklet issued free by the Royal National Institute for the Deaf, 'TV and Radio Adaptors and the Loop System'. Most voluntary societies will arrange for radio sets to be repaired, and a number have volunteers who will service these sets free.

Television
In the autumn of 1980 a new TV sound receiver was produced to enable blind people to have a set on which they could listen to the sound content of TV programmes, but for which no TV licence need

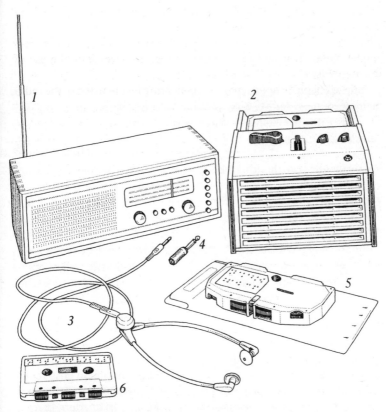

1 Press-button radio, issued by British Wireless for the Blind Fund
2 Talking Book machine
3 Stethophones (issued free by B.W.B.F.) which can be plugged into radio and also with aid of jackplug (4) into talking book machine, to ensure undisturbed listening
5 Talking Book cassette which can only be played on special machine (2).
6 Cassette issued by Calibre library which can be played on any standard cassette machine

be paid, as it receives no pictures! Some blind people have claimed that its sound quality is better than that of a conventional TV set. The receiver is easy to use once it has been tuned; a simple push button operation is all that is needed to switch channels. But the set can only be used in areas where UHF television programmes are available.

The sound receiver can be bought from the RNIB for £50. It is being produced by Marconi Hillend, a Youth Opportunities Workshop in Fife, whose prime function is to train unemployed school leavers in electronics, so that they can then proceed to jobs in open industry. This model is an adaptation of the first television sound receiver made for the RNIB by Decca; although it is no longer being produced, Decca will still undertake repairs and service for their sets. Contact Spares and Service Department, *Decca Radio and Television Ltd, Stanmore Industrial Estate, Bridgnorth, Shropshire (tel. Bridgnorth (07462) 4121*.

Blind people who have an ordinary television set get a reduction of £1.25 on their television licence. The local authority will supply a certificate of blindness which should be taken to the post office when paying for the licence and then kept to use again in future years.

Recorded books
There is a vast range of English language books specially recorded for blind people. The British Talking Book Service has over 3,600 titles; its American counterpart, the Library of Congress National Library Service for the Blind and Physically Handicapped, has 30,000 titles. There is a Student Tape Library in London which has about 4,000 titles and its counterpart in New York, Recording for the Blind, has about 50,000 educational books on cassette. In addition there are other tape libraries, on both sides of the Atlantic, which are adding new recordings to their lists every week. It is unfortunate that it is impossible for any blind person to take advantage of this range of recorded books unless he or she has access to three different tape recorders or playback machines. Both the British Talking Book Service and the US Library Service for the Blind and Physically Handicapped record their books on to cassettes that can only be played on special machines made available by the respective libraries to their blind listeners, but the machines and tapes are not interchangeable; both the American and the British libraries are bound by the terms of their agreements with publishers to reproduce their books in limited

editions and in non-commercially available form and unfortunately the two libraries have chosen different ways of achieving the same end. As a result any blind person who wished to borrow both the English and the American recorded books would need to have two different tape machines, and neither of these machines could also play the books recorded by Calibre, or most of the recorded newspapers or magazines which are available in so many localities as these are usually produced on standard compact cassettes which have to be played back on an ordinary cassette recorder. It is therefore very important for all those choosing recorded books to be certain that they have the correct playback equipment.

The problems caused to the blind reader by these different systems have been a subject of concern to Arthur Wilson, the Director of the Foundation for Audio Research, for a number of years. It is part of the Foundation's policy to make available to blind people in Britain audio machines which can reproduce books made from master recordings used in all the current systems. To this end, the Foundation has been involved in the creation of an Audio Reading Trust, with this specific objective in view (see page 169 for more details about the Foundation).

Mr Wilson points out that there are, in addition to blind and partially-sighted people, many others who are unable to read because of various handicaps, e.g. dyslexia or physical inability to hold a book or turn its pages. He estimates that, including illiterates, there are about two million print-handicapped people in Britain and the Audio Reading Trust's long-term aim is to produce its own Audio books, which can be distributed through the public library system or sold at a reasonable price. These Audio books would be recorded on compact cassette, but at a much lower speed than normal, so it will be possible to have eight hours on a C90 cassette, and thus enable an average novel to be recorded on to two such cassettes. The Trust is planning to manufacture the special playback machine needed for those Audio books; but unlike other such specialist machines, these would also be able to play cassettes recorded at standard speeds. The Trust hopes that the first of these Audio books and machines will become available late in 1982.

British Talking Book Library

This is the service most widely used by blind people in Britain. In 1981, over 54,000 belonged to it. The choice of books, which are recorded by professionals, ranges over standard favourites as reflected in public library loans. It is mostly fiction. About 350 titles are added each year, though it is hoped to increase this to about 400 annually in future. But this is only a tiny fraction of the 27,000 books published annually in Britain. The Talking Book Service also includes a small selection of children's books.

The talking book machines are issued to any registered blind person, and also to any other visually handicapped person who can supply a certificate, signed by an ophthalmologist, stating that they have defective reading vision (generally N.12 or worse with spectacles). The playback machines are specially designed so that they can easily be worked by totally blind people. The Talking Book machine cannot be bought: it is available on loan to members who pay an annual subscription (in 1981 this was £12). Many of the 54,000 members have their subscription paid either by their local authority or their local voluntary organisation.

Books are chosen from the catalogue, a copy of which is sent to every new reader. As the catalogue is only updated after every 1,000 new titles, additions to the Talking Book library are listed in the RNIB's monthly journal *New Beacon* or in the *Braille Monthly Announcements*. On joining, a member is asked to send in a list of about thirty requests, and as far as possible the Talking Book Service tries to ensure that all readers have a book of their choice sent regularly. All selection and despatch procedures have been computerised, and the Talking Book Service claims that the computer has been programmed so that a reader should never be without a book, provided that books are returned promptly.

It is possible to listen to talking books without disturbing others in the same room by using either stethophones (price £4.50) or headphones (price £5.50) which are both available from the Library. People confined to bed can get pillow phones to special order. It is also possible to buy from the Library a jack plug adaptor (price 75p) so that the stethophones issued by the Wireless for the Blind Fund for their radio (see page 163) can be used on a talking book machine. It is also possible to get a limited number of variable speed talking book machines from the Talking Book Library.

For people who have additional handicaps, such as arthritic hands, which make it difficult to operate the playback machines it is possible to get adaptations which might enable them to operate their machines unaided. These are extended controls for the on/off knob or the track-change button, which give more leverage and a simple remote control switch can be added to enable a bed-ridden person to switch the machine on or off. Details from *The British Talking Book Service for the Blind, Mount Pleasant, Wembley, Middlesex HA0 1RR (tel. 01-903 6666)*, to whom also all new applications for membership should be sent.

Calibre
This is a lending library of books recorded on to standard compact cassettes which can be played on any ordinary cassette player. In 1981, its catalogue included nearly 2,000 titles, among them several hundred children's titles. The organisers try to record new fiction and base their selections on the best seller lists. The library tries as far as possible to ensure that all their members receive tapes within a day or two of returning their books; and although the books are recorded in their own homes by volunteer readers (many of them, however, are professional actors or actresses who give their services free) the quality of recording is very good. Membership of Calibre is free to individuals who are able to supply a doctor's certificate stating their inability to read printed books. Calibre also offers group membership for £30 a year to schools, hospitals and other institutions such as toy libraries, which allows them to get four books at a time. Applications to *Calibre, Aylesbury, Buckinghamshire HP20 1HU (tel. Aylesbury (0296) 32339)*.

American libraries
The American equivalent of the British Talking Book Library is the Library for Blind and Physically Handicapped; it has a far wider range of books – 30,000 titles of which 4,000 are children's books. The recordings are on four-track cassettes, played at the very low speed of $^{15}/_{16}$ inches per second (ips), which means that each cassette covers six hours of recording. This is known as the 'Library of Congress' format.

It is possible for individual readers, through a library, to borrow books from libraries in other countries through the inter-library loan scheme, and this could theoretically apply to tape as well as to print libraries. When the idea of borrowing from the US Library for the Blind and Physically Handicapped was mooted on an *In Touch* programme in the autumn of 1980 there was an enthusiastic response. But the Director of the US Library stated that he felt it would 'violate the spirit of inter-library loan' if more than fifty books at a time were

167

loaned: and The British Talking Book Service, faced with a much larger demand from blind people, felt that it would not be practical or appropriate for them to attempt to restrict or select applications. Thus there is no possibility of exchanges between the US Library for the Blind and Physically Handicapped and blind people in Britain, who have the appropriate playback machine, through the Talking Book Service. However it is possible for blind people in this country to make use of the extensive tape library (over 50,000 titles) stocked by Recording for the Blind, Inc. This library was set up to serve the needs of blind students, but is willing to lend to any blind person. Details, and application forms, from *Recording for the Blind, Inc., 215 East 58th Street, New York, NY 10022*. All tapes in this library are also recorded in the 'Library of Congress' format.

The New York Jewish Guild for the Blind:
Despite its title this is not a sectarian organisation and its taped library reflects current American tastes. The Librarian is happy to consider applications from Britain. The recordings are on standard cassettes, and unlike those in the other libraries listed here, some of the readings have been dramatised. Full details from *Bruce Massis, Librarian, Jewish Guild for the Blind, 15 West 65th Street, New York, NY 10023*.

Student Tape Library
The situation for borrowers from the RNIB's student tape library is complicated by the fact that although all new recordings are made on to C90 cassettes, which can be played on any standard cassette machine, the majority of their titles are still on Talking Book cassettes, which require the special playback equipment. However, despite its title, the Student Tape Library is available for use by anyone interested in serious reading. New recordings will only be made for full-time students or teachers, but anyone registered blind or with a suitable certificate from an ophthalmologist stating inability to read print, can make use of the books. The books are read by volunteers, mostly specialists in the subjects concerned, which range from statistics to politics, history to theology. For full details contact *Helma Urquhart, Librarian, Braille House, 338-46 Goswell Road, London EC1V 7JE*.

Talking newspapers

Talking newspaper groups produce taped versions of local newspapers and distribute these weekly or fortnightly to blind, partially sighted and severely handicapped people. This is a rapidly growing movement with some 300 established projects in 1981, and at least a hundred more in various stages of development. Some talking newspapers also provide magazines and personal tape services. The co-ordinating body is the Talking Newspaper Association of the United Kingdom, whose aim is to make a taped newspaper available to every visually handicapped person in the country. Information on existing groups and help with starting new ones is available from *Jo Deaper, Chairman, Talking Newspaper Association of the United Kingdom (TNAUK), 4 Southgate Street, Winchester, Hampshire (tel. Winchester (0962) 65570)*.

There is no national tape newspaper, but extracts from national newspapers are recorded by some local talking newspapers. Further information from the Talking Newspaper Association. Extracts from the *Sunday Times* and articles of topical scientific interest are available from the *Tape Service of the Cultural Society for the Disabled, 10 Warwick Row, London SW1*.

'Soundaround'

'Soundaround' is a tape magazine which aims to give a monthly regional round-up of news concerning the visually handicapped as well as providing a general interest tape magazine. It is available free from *Nigel Verbeek, 61 Church Road, Barnes, London SW13 (tel. 01-741 3332)*.

Tape recorders

There is a wide range of tape recorders available and there is no reason why a blind person should not just seek the advice of a local shop. The RNIB does make a limited number of tape recorders available at concession prices to blind people, but they do not operate an after-sales service. The best source of advice on all matters relating to tape recorders and other sound equipment for blind people is Arthur E. Wilson OBE, a retired senior civil servant, who in 1976 set up the Foundation for Audio Research and Services to Blind People, with the aim of providing sound equipment exactly suited to blind people's needs. The Foundation is not geared to do a *Which?*-style comparison

169

and analysis of all the many recorders on the market, but it can offer advice on the kind of machine that is likely to be of value. A blind student's needs are not likely to be served properly by the simple machine with easy controls which is all that an elderly blind person may need to listen to a talking newspaper or a tape letter. Nor would such an elderly person necessarily want some of the more sophisticated equipment available from the Foundation. Among the items stocked by the Foundation are machines which will play tapes recorded in the 'Library of Congress' format, and variable speed tape recorders, on which it is possible to play back tapes, without pitch distortions, either at half-speed, or up to two and a half times as fast, as the speed at which it was originally recorded. The Foundation has also introduced the facility of tone-indexing on to many of the tape recorders it sells. Tone-indexing is the blind person's alternative to the counters with which a sighted person using a tape recorder can locate the right place on a tape. Any tape recorder which has the facility of cue/review enables the user to hear the high-pitched chatter of recordings as the tape is fast-wound in either direction. With tone-indexing a 'bleep' signal can be put on the tape during recording to act as a sign for a new chapter, beginning of a new recipe, different set of telephone numbers, and so on, and when the tape is subsequently fast wound the 'bleep' can be clearly heard and act as a place finder. As well as selling recorders with tone-indexing facilities, the Foundation will consider adapting any cassette recorders which have cue/review facilities. A catalogue listing their full range of equipment is available (price 25p) from the Foundation.

Spoken word recordings
Obviously the whole range of recorded music is open to blind people. There is also a wide range of spoken word records and cassettes which can be a source of pleasure to those unable to read print and which often can be borrowed from public libraries. The magazine, *The Gramophone*, issues an annual spoken word catalogue, which details the vast range available. It includes poetry, play recordings, Bible-readings and miscellanies. Details from *General Gramophone Publications, 177/179 Kenton Road, Harrow, Middlesex HA3 0HA (tel. 01-907 4476)*.

Those who wish to buy spoken word cassettes may find it worth while getting in touch with some of the mail order firms that specialise in this field, as record shops and firms such as Boots or W.H. Smith usually only have a very limited selection. All the mail order firms named below will give some discounts to blind customers and will send catalogues on request. Talktapes also offers special interest lists on subjects including poetry, drama and humour, science fiction and children's books. Full details from *Talktapes, 13 Croftdown Road, London NW5 1EL (tel. 01-485 9981)*.

A wide range of spoken word cassettes are listed in a catalogue available free from *Record and Tape Sales, Newmarket Road, Bury St Edmunds, Suffolk 1P33 3YB (tel. Bury St Edmunds (0284) 68011)*.

Other firms dealing in spoken word cassettes are *Chivers Book Sales Ltd, 93-100 Locksbrook Road, Bath B41 3HB (tel. Bath (0225) 316872)* and *Audio Visual Library Services Ltd, 10-12 Powdrake Road, Grangemouth, Stirlingshire FK3 9UT (tel. Grangemouth (032 44) 71521/2)*.

Tape-recording services
There are a number of tape services designed specially for the needs of visually-handicapped people.

Free Tape Recorded Library for the Blind: Ron Hall, who is totally blind and worked as a telephonist until he retired in 1980, has in his spare time recorded a series of over 400 programmes. They last from thirty to ninety minutes and range in subject from visits to places such as Westminster Abbey or the Bluebell Railway to long interviews with personalities, among them Prince Philip. Mr Hall has also made programmes with less well-known people; his tapes include the reminiscences of a centenarian, a candid interview with a prostitute and a series with a group of gipsies. Some of his most popular programmes are accounts of his own holiday travels. Mr Hall cannot undertake to supply individual requests for particular programmes, but will try to provide his listeners with something suitable every week. All programmes are recorded on cassette or five-inch spools at 3¾ ips and people can join the library on payment of £1, after which all tapes are sent free. Details from *Ron Hall, 26 Laggan Road, Maidenhead, Berkshire SL6 7JZ (tel. Maidenhead (0628) 20014)*.

Reading services: Charles Cadwell manages the Tape Recording Service for the Blind, primarily aimed at recording on to tape any printed material for people unable to read for themselves. His volunteer readers are prepared to tackle anything from an instruction leaflet for

171

a piece of domestic equipment to a full-length book, if it is not available elsewhere. He prefers not to record material of a political or religious nature. A number of magazines for blind readers, including the RNIB's *New Beacon* and *Viewpoint*, the journal of the National Federation of the Blind, are regularly recorded, as is the *In Touch* quarterly bulletin. In addition, Mr Cadwell produces two bi-monthly tape magazines, one of which is particularly geared to women's interests. He can also supply some elementary language courses, a course of touch typing and a taped catalogue of the Talking Book Service. Material is sent free if requests are accompanied by tape or cassette for recording; otherwise the only charge is the price of a tape or cassette and any expenses the reader may incur (these are invariably minimal). Details from *Charles Cadwell, MBE, 48 Fairfax Road, Farnborough, Hampshire GU14 8JP (tel. Farnborough (0252) 47943)*.

A very similar service is operated by another blind man, George Causey, whose Tape Programmes for Blind People aims to supplement the work done by Mr Cadwell. Full details from *Mr Causey, Agorita, 31 Fortescue Road, Paignton, Devon TQ3 2BY (tel. Paignton (0803) 522873)*.

Another reading service is run by Mrs Audrey Artus, whose volunteer readers include a number who will undertake recordings in French, German, Spanish and Italian. The ADA Reading Service will record material of any length. Details from *Mrs Artus, 12 Renhold Road, Wilden, Bedfordshire (tel. Bedford (0234) 771693)*.

Certain local voluntary societies for the blind will record material on request for blind people in their area. These include:

Scotland: *Resource Centre for the Blind, 276 St Vincent Street, Glasgow G2 5RP (tel. 041-248 5811)*.

Wales: *North Wales Society for the Blind, 325 High Street, Bangor, Gwynedd LL57 1YB (tel. Bangor (0248) 53604)*.

Midlands: *Birmingham Royal Institution for the Blind, 49 Oak Court Road, Harborne, Birmingham (tel. 021-427 2248)* (a personal reader, rather than a tape recording, is provided on a one to one basis).

Other voluntary societies for the blind might well be able to help with reading, if they are asked, and it might also be worth enquiring if the people involved in the local talking newspaper can help.

Express Reading Service: Since 1977 Mrs Wendy Davies has run a free fast reading service for print material which is urgently required for work, study or leisure purposes. She guarantees to record and send back a tape by return of post, but the service can only undertake one hour's worth of recording per day for any individual: with larger items, the service will try to return a tape a day until the reading is completed. The Centre can record items at standard, half-speed and in the American Library of Congress format, and will also undertake to add tone-indexing. The Centre was set up under the aegis of the Foundation for Audio Research, but in June 1981 the RNIB took it over and plans to open another centre in Cheshire to expand the service. Full details of service from *Mrs Davies, 79 High Street, Tarporley, Cheshire (tel. Tarporley (082 93) 2115 or 2729).*

Devotional material on tape
St Cecilia's Guild for the Blind was established about thirty years ago to make available Christian and Catholic literature for the blind. It has a large library of devotional literature and readings available on cassettes. Full details from the librarian – *Miss C. Beard, 21 Elvin Crescent, Rottingdean, East Sussex BN2 7FF (tel. Brighton (0273) 36892).*

The Torch Trust for the Blind has a stock of missionary books, scriptures and Christian magazines on tape. Many of its books are now available on talking book cassettes. Details from *Torch House, Hallaton, Market Harborough, Leicestershire LE16 8UJ (tel. Hallaton (085 889) 301).*

Tape recordings of sermons, lessons and other Christian teachings are available on loan from the Worldwide Evangelical Tape Fellowship. Full details from the secretary, *Mike Cox, 99 Pilgrims Way, Kemsing, near Sevenoaks, Kent (tel. Sevenoaks (0732) 61447).*

The Taped Ministry can supply, on cassette, recorded versions of all the books in the New Testament on loan, or for sale. It also has a tape library of Christian literature. Details from *Roland G. Jones, Hilltop, 137 Fairwater Grove West, Llandaff, Cardiff CF5 2JP (tel. Cardiff (0222) 568359).*

The Muriel Braddick Foundation provides housebound and handicapped people with specially prepared cassette recordings geared to the specific interest of the recipient, who can where necessary also be given an easily handled cassette recorder. Mrs Muriel Braddick MBE, the founder, is a committed Christian who is blind and suffers from a progressive muscular disease. Full details about the service offered by the foundation from its headquarters at *14 Teign Street, Teignmouth, Devon (tel. Teignmouth (06267) 6214).*

Specialist tape services

A fortnightly cassette of material of interest to lawyers is circulated by the Society of Blind Lawyers. The material, selected by a solicitor, covers law reports and readings of articles from law journals. Annual subscription £15. Details from *Jeremy Browne, 33 Cornfields, Box-moor, Hemel Hempstead, Hertfordshire (tel. Hemel Hempstead (0442) 47627)*.

A tape version of the journal of the British Association of Social Workers, *Social Work Today*, can be obtained from *Michael Brace, 80 Elms Farm Road, Hornchurch, Essex RM12 5RD (tel. Hornchurch (040 24) 56832)*.

The British Computer Association of the Blind produces a fort-nightly cassette, suitable for playback on Talking Book machines. It contains articles from all the leading British data processing papers and journals, including those of the British Computer Society. Enquiries to *The Secretary, British Computer Association of the Blind, BCM Box 950, London WC1V 6XX (tel. Gerald Neal, Guildford (0483) 68121, ext. 373)*.

Many sighted tape recordists are only too pleased to do some recording for a visually handicapped person. The Federation of British Recordists and Clubs publishes a quarterly '*News and Views*' and would be happy to include appeals for help in this magazine. Enquiries to *J. Hicks, 32 Markfield, Courtwood Lane, Addington, Surrey CR0 9HH (tel. 01-657 0505)*.

Tape correspondence clubs

The tape equivalent of pen-pals is available to any blind person who owns a tape recorder or cassette player. A number of tape correspon-dence clubs will put anyone interested in touch with suitable contacts. One of the best known is Worldwide Tapetalk, *Secretary, Charles L. Towers, 35 The Gardens, West Harrow, Middlesex HA1 4HE (tel. 01-863 0706)*. The annual subscription is £3 plus £1 initial enrolment fee, for which applicants get a membership card, a useful booklet of hints on recording messages, the club magazine and an up-to-date directory of members to enable the new member to get in touch straightaway with a suitable correspondent.

There is also the Chatterbox Recording Club, *Secretary, Dick Arm-strong, 1 Chestnut Drive, Holme-on-Spalding, Moor, York YO4 4HW (tel. Market Weighton (0696) 60403)*. This has special interest groups such as classical music, jazz and a ladies' section. A directory of members is sent to everyone on joining, so that they can select their 'tape-pals'.

In 1979, a blind lady, Mrs Muriel Baker, set up her own tape club designed to help other housebound blind people to find friends. She offers a free service: anyone who wants to join should send a cassette listing their personal details and interests to *Mrs Baker, Setts Wood Farm, Leigh Green, Tenterden, Kent*.

There is also a Tape Friends Club run by *Mrs Mary Thomas, 8 Leasowes Road, Kings Heath, Birmingham B14 7AU (tel. 021 449 6923)*. Send cassette giving name, address and interests to Mrs Thomas.

Another Birmingham based group, Tape Programmes for the Blind, which is run by Squadron-Leader Maurice Chambers, circulates 'round-robin' tapes to small groups of people, each of whom is expected to add half an hour to the recording. For details write to *Kingsmead, Blackfirs Lane, Marston Green, Birmingham B37 7JE (tel. 021 779 3202)*.

People who are enthusiastic to try their hand at more ambitious forms of recording might like to know that the British Amateur Tape Recording Contest presents a special award to the best recording made by a handicapped person, and over the years blind people have won this as well as other awards in this annual event. Full details from *John Bradley, 33 Fairlawnes, Malden Road, Wallington, Surrey SM6 8BG (tel. 01-669 2982)*.

Radio amateurs

Many blind people get a great deal of enjoyment out of operating short-wave radio sets. Nearly half the members of the Radio Amateur Invalid and Blind Club are visually handicapped. The club will put blind amateur radio enthusiasts in touch with local representatives and radio clubs who can help them with the initial installation of equipment as well as with any necessary repairs and maintenance. Blind people wishing to obtain a transmitting licence can get their study material transcribed into braille or on to tape, and the Post Office is prepared to allow blind candidates unable to write or type to take their examination orally. Membership is free for blind people. Details from the honorary secretary, *Mrs Frances Woolley, 9 Rannoch Court, Adelaide Road, Surbiton, Surrey KT6 4TE (tel. 01-390 2803)*.

Another society for blind radio 'hams' is run by St Dunstan's. Only the war-blinded are admitted to full membership, but other visually-handicapped people are eligible for associate membership. Details from *E.C. John, 52 Broadway Avenue, Wallasey, Merseyside, L45 6TD (tel. Liverpool (051) 638 5514).*

A self-help organisation known as BRAAGIS (Blind Radio Amateur Auditory Gimmicks Information Service) has been set up by Peter Jones, a blind electronics enthusiast. For details contact him at *69 Prospect Road, Bradway, Sheffield S17 4JB (tel. Sheffield (0742) 309199).*

★   *Slip different numbers of rubber bands over cassettes to distinguish the lengths – e.g. 1 rubber band for C60s, 2 rubber bands for C90s.*
(Muriel Baker, Tenterden)

★   *You can balance a cassette on your finger to tell which side is heavier and so know which way to insert it into the machine.*
(David Scott Blackhall)

★   *Use a blob of Hi-Marks to tell side A of your cassettes.*
(Hannah Wright)

4 Leisure

The leisure time interests of visually-handicapped people are as varied as those of the rest of the community. Wherever possible, many want to join ordinary local clubs and societies rather than seek special facilities for the blind. It is often more appropriate to help the visually handicapped with transport to clubs of their choice, where they can, if necessary, use adapted equipment (braille playing cards, for instance) rather than segregate blind people into a special club.

The British Association for Sporting and Recreational Activities of the Blind (BASRAB) was set up in 1975 to help blind and partially sighted people in all matters relating to leisure time activities. The Association hopes to encourage blind people to participate in a wide range of sports and recreation in the community, but it will also help to provide special facilities where these are needed. BASRAB also plans to act as a pressure group to ensure that the needs of the blind are taken into account when sports and recreational facilities are planned in the community. The Association is anxious to help any blind or partially sighted people with any problems regarding sports or recreation and also hopes to establish a central register of information. For all details contact the chairman *Frank McFarlane, 11 Ovolo Road, Liverpool L13 3DR (tel. 051-220 2516)*. In addition, the RNIB has a Sports and Recreation Officer who should be able to provide helpful information about the provision made for any particular sport or hobby.

Angling

Many people continue to enjoy fishing despite poor sight, and totally blind fishermen have even won cups in local contests. The National Anglers Council say that most local clubs are very sympathetic to the needs of blind anglers, and will be pleased to help them if at all possible. Probably any local fishing tackle shop will give addresses of local clubs, but in case of difficulties the *National Anglers Council, 11 Cowgate, Peterborough PE1 1LZ (tel. Peterborough (0733) 54084)*, will supply the address of the nearest club.

The Council has also produced a useful booklet, *Guide to Fishing Facilities for Disabled Anglers*, which is obtainable from them for £1, including postage. There is also a braille edition of *Teach Yourself*

Fishing available in two volumes (catalogue nos 25149/50) from the RNIB at the concessionary price of 80p. Blind anglers may like to try out Newark needle floats which the inventor, Walter Bower, claims to be particularly suitable for the blind. Instead of the traditional arrangement of separate float and different sizes of lead weights, Mr Bower has designed a combined float and weighting system, which can be easily attached to the fishing line. Mr Bower claims that it is impossible to tangle the system when casting. Newark needle floats are on sale at Woolworths (not fishing tackle shops) and cost £1.35 for a set of four.

Art

Quite a number of visually handicapped people successfully do art work which is tactile (for example collage) but at least one totally blind person, Flight Lieutenant Gordon Stent, who lost his sight on active service in the Second World War, has proved that it is possible to paint successfully without sight. He has evolved special techniques for painting with such success that his work has been hung in open exhibitions with sighted artists, without anyone being aware of his handicap. Mr Stent has basically devised two different techniques: the first uses a plastic needle or similar instrument to make the outline markings on art paper; this can be felt by the tips of the fingers, and is coloured with an oil-based crayon which does not smudge and gives a fine, polished finish. The second technique requires more exacting control and uses oil paint soluble in turpentine. Mr Stent is willing to teach his techniques to any interested blind or visually handicapped person. Enquiries to him at *40 Surrey Road, Bournemouth, Dorset BH4 9BX (tel. Bournemouth (0202) 761905)*.

A drawing aid for the blind has been invented by a designer, Ron van der Meer. It consists of a piece of rubber-coated board which has an indented frame around three sides with notches to indicate centimetres and a movable T-square. An ordinary piece of paper can be put on the board and a blind person exerting only slight pressure with ballpoint pen, pencil or waxed crayon can produce a tangible design. The frame and T-square enable it to be used also for diagrams or maps. Mr van der Meer has taught a number of blind pupils at Chorleywood College to use the board with very pleasing results; an exhibition of their work was held at the Whitechapel Gallery in 1975. Unfortunately the board is not produced commercially, but Mr van der Meer would be happy to explain the details of the design to anyone wanting to make one. Address: *143 Marlborough Road, Langley, Berkshire SL3 7JG (tel. Slough (0753) 41257).*

Bingo

A number of organisations, as well as individuals, have designed their own versions of bingo, played with boards and markers that can be used even by totally blind people. These bingo boards are produced only in small quantities for the use of local groups and are not generally available.

Some clubs for blind people play a version of bingo based on dominoes. One method of play invented by the Cleveland and South Durham Institute for the Blind is as follows. There are four players to each table; each player has seven dominoes. A caller sits at the top table and has a full set of dominoes, which are shuffled thoroughly. Domino 6/4 is always called first to start the game and every person who has that number places it in the middle of the table. The first person to have seven dominoes out calls 'house' and the caller checks the dominoes. There is another version of 'domino-bingo' invented by the Brighton Society for the Welfare of the Blind. Players sit two to a table and one set of dominoes (double blank to double six) is allowed to each table. Each player draws nine dominoes, leaving ten in the box. The same nine may be retained for each game, or the set may be shuffled and redealt. The player places the dominoes face upwards immediately in front of him and turns each one over when that number is called. The caller has a complete set of dominoes which are shuffled and placed face downward on the table. They are picked up at random and, after being called, placed to one side in numerical order so that checking is easy. The caller continues until a player has had all his or her numbers called, and when this happens the player cries 'bingo'.

These bingo games are designed for groups of blind players, but obviously are unsuitable for use in an ordinary bingo hall. John Broughton, a blind man in Lincoln, has designed a bingo board with braille and ordinary markings, in which round-headed rivets are put into countersunk holes to mark the card. With the permission of local managements he and other blind people have been playing with these cards at ordinary bingo halls, and Mr Broughton reports that several blind players, using his cards, have not only been able to keep up with sighted players but have won on several occasions. Mr Broughton claims that he has had over 2,000 requests for his board from blind individuals and organisations catering for their needs, but he has to date not succeeded in getting a manufacturer interested in taking on its production. Enquiries about the cards (accompanied by a stamped addressed envelope) should be addressed to him at *22 Carlton Grove, Ermine East, Lincoln LN2 2EA (tel. Lincoln (0522) 24780)*.

Birds

Bird fanciers might like to follow the example of a totally blind man, Jed Jackson, who has for nearly thirty years successfully bred and raced pigeons. He will be glad to advise any other blind person interested in following this sport. Address: *5 New Road, Durrington, Worthing, Sussex BN13 3JG (tel. Worthing (0903) 64087)*.

Bowling

So many visually-handicapped people continue to enjoy the game of bowls that a National Association of Visually Handicapped Bowlers was formally constituted in October 1976. It sets out to promote interest in the welfare of visually handicapped bowlers, providing where possible teaching amenities and financial help, and acts as a liaison with other national and international organisations. The main events of the year are the three open tournaments for visually handicapped bowlers held at Hastings, Lowestoft and Weston-super-Mare. In July 1980 the Association held its first national tournament in Leicester, and it is hoped to make this an annual event. Addresses of local clubs, some useful hints on coaching new players and any other information about the Association can be obtained from the president, *Mrs M. Dennis, 23 Bodnant Avenue, Leicester LE5 5RB (tel. Leicester (0533) 736420)*.

The Scottish Association of Blind Bowlers was formed some years ago and bowling enthusiasts in Scotland can obtain information from the honorary secretary and treasurer, *Mr R. Wm Mackie, 4 Coates Crescent, Edinburgh EH3 7AP (tel. Edinburgh (031)225 6381)*.

A booklet *How to Coach Blind Bowlers* can be obtained free from the *Tourism and Recreation Department, Hastings Borough Council, 4 Robertson Terrace, Hastings, E. Sussex TN34 1JE (tel. Hastings (0424) 424242)*.

Ten-pin bowling
This is also a popular sport. In some parts of the country, groups of blind people have got together and hold matches against other blind and sighted teams. Advice on how to start such a group will be supplied on request by the *West Sussex Association for the Blind, 26 Southgate, Chichester, Sussex PO19 1ES (tel. Chichester (0243) 788333).*

Card games
Ordinary playing cards marked in braille are available from RNIB, which also produces brailled cards for Happy Families, Lexicon and Whot. All are suitable for sighted and blind people playing together, as apart from the braille symbols the cards are standard in design and size. Because frequent handling can erase the braille dots, or make them less easy to feel, a new system of plastic coating has been designed to increase durability and standard playing cards treated in this way are available at a slightly higher price.

Playing cards and Lexicon cards and smaller playing cards for Patience, which are embossed in Moon type, are available from the Moon branch of the RNIB. It is not necessary to be fluent braille or Moon readers to use these cards – only a knowledge of the alphabet is required.

Other special aids for card players include a Patience board, which is suitable for use only with special packs of braille Patience cards, also supplied by the RNIB. Bridge players might like to know that a totally blind man, Bert Ward, works as an instructor in local evening classes and he will be happy to advise visually handicapped bridge players on any difficulties they may have. His address is *9 Wynford Terrace, Leeds LS16 6HU (tel. Leeds (0532) 674812).*

Large print playing cards
There are a number of different types of large print playing cards. The Society for the Blind in Dumfries and Galloway produces a pack of cards with a large index number in the top right hand corner and a large symbol with initial in the corner of the card. A pack of these cards costs 30p obtainable direct from the Society, *24 Catherine Street, Dumfries DG1 1HZ (tel. Dumfries (0387) 3927).*

Waddingtons produce Easy-to-See cards which are of normal size, but have extra large symbols and numerals. These are available in some shops (Woolworths, John Menzies) for £1.65 a pack, but they are obtainable more cheaply (£1.04 a pack) to personal shoppers only at the RNIB shop at 224 Great Portland Street, London W1N 6AA. They can also be obtained direct from the *Waddington Playing Card Co. Ltd, Wakefield Road, Leeds LS10 3TP (tel. Leeds (0532) 712233)*. Add 30p a pack for postage and packing.

Piatnik also produce large-print playing cards obtainable from good stationers or large department stores, or by post from *Benno Products, Playing Cards Distributors, 27 Little Russell Street, London WC1A 2HN (tel. 01-405 7030)*. Their 'Large Index' normal-sized cards cost 91p a pack (plus 19p postage) and the 'Kingsbridge Bill Boards', which are jumbo-sized cards, are £4.45 a pack (plus 58p postage).

Chess

Special chess sets for blind players, including a pocket set, are available from the RNIB; all the white chess pieces have a point at the top so that they can be easily distinguished from the black by touch, and all the chess pieces have small pegs at the bottom so that they can be plugged into holes on the chessboard. The black squares on the board are raised, and the white slightly sunk, to distinguish them for blind players. There is a Braille Chess Association which organises a biennial chess championship for the blind, in conjunction with the British Chess Federation. The Association, which welcomes all players from beginners to experts, also organises weekend tournaments and postal chess games between members both in Britain and abroad. Full details from the secretary, *Mr J. Horrocks, 59 Sefton Street, London SW15 1NA (tel. 01-785 9844)*.

A comprehensive tape library of chess material is available from the Braille Chess Association; and the American chess magazine *En Passant* can be obtained from the *Tape Recording Service for the Blind*.

Cricket

Blind cricket enthusiasts have formed a National Cricket League and matches are played throughout the season.

The game of cricket played by teams of blind and partially sighted people bears little resemblance to test cricket. It is played with a football, to give blind players a larger target to aim for. So that the ball will rattle, it is filled with lead shot of the type used by fishermen.

Rules are also adapted. The ball must bounce at least once before reaching a partially sighted batsman, and at least twice for a totally blind batsman, so that he can detect its direction. The bowler must say 'ready' and then play. Totally blind fieldsmen may take a catch off one bounce. Teams are made up of seven partially sighted and four totally blind players. The game has to be played without too much extraneous noise, noise level being the equivalent of light for the sighted cricketer. Cricket is becoming an increasingly popular game for visually handicapped sportsmen. Standards of play may be nowhere near professional, but participants and spectators can still enjoy the involvement and the fun of competition.

Addresses of cricket clubs for the blind can be obtained either from the Recreation Officer at the Royal National Institute for the Blind or *George Simmons, 248 Mottingham Road, Eltham, London SE9 (tel. 01-851 1840).*

Dancing

Blind people who would like to take up dancing may find that there are suitable classes run by local adult education institutes. There may also be courses run specifically for blind people. Some local voluntary societies for the blind run classes. But there is no reason why a visually handicapped student should not join ordinary classes together with sighted students. A check by the *In Touch* office indicated that applications from blind as well as other handicapped students would be treated sympathetically by adult education institutes, which would try to help them follow the courses of their choice if at all possible.

Drama

Participation in amateur dramatics can be a valuable activity for visually handicapped people, not only as a new interest but also as a way of restoring confidence in those who have lost their sight. Quite a number of visually handicapped people have joined ordinary local drama groups. Apart from the classes run in adult education centres, there are also numerous amateur dramatic groups and details of the nearest are obtainable from the *National Operatic and Dramatic Association, 1 Crestfield Street, London EC1H 8AT (tel. 01-837 5655).*

There are also several exclusively blind drama groups including a very active group run by the Jewish Blind Society; and The Venturers in West London (for details contact *Mrs P. Bailey, Flat 5, 43 Avenue Gardens, Acton, London W3 8HB (tel. 01-992 9921)).*

In Leeds there is a Blind Drama Group run by the social services department of the city council. Details from *Mr B. Naylor, Social Services, West Division, Redcourt, Church Road, Armley, Leeds 12.*

Since 1975 there have been annual residential drama courses for blind people, as well as weekend workshops to train anyone interested in setting up local amateur groups for the blind. Details of these activities can be obtained from *Judy Fairclough, 37 Tappesfield Road, Nunhead, London SE15 3EY (tel. 01-732 2356).*

Esperanto

There is a special association for blind Esperantists, which aims to spread knowledge of the language among the blind and to further contact between blind Esperantists at home and abroad. The association runs a braille correspondence course and tape recordings of pronunciation and readings from Esperanto textbooks are also available. Full details from the honorary secretary, *Miss S. Yates, 4 Drinkwater Close, Eastleigh, Hampshire.*

Football

A number of football clubs make special arrangements for a limited number of blind spectators. Clubs with facilities for relaying match commentaries to patients in local hospitals often allow blind people to sit in the commentary box or adjoining stands where they can hear the commentary on headphones. Some clubs issue free passes to local blind people; details about individual club arrangements can be obtained on inquiry from the local club secretary. Details of football results, league tables and fixtures are available weekly throughout the season in braille from the Scottish Braille Press and in Moon from the Moon Branch of the RNIB.

Five-a-side football

A national league for five-a-side football was launched in January 1980. Clubs or groups of blind or partially sighted people prepared to form a team can obtain details from *Mr R. Goulden, 1 Malvern Close, Prestwich, Manchester M25 5PH (tel. 061-798 9137, evenings only).*

Gardening

This is one of the most popular leisure time pursuits for visually handicapped people and the Southern and Western Regional Association for the Blind have shown a particular interest in promoting activities for blind gardeners. The Association organises an annual residential weekend course for blind gardeners, as well as seminars for sighted people on gardening with the blind. For more details contact *Brian Eccles* at the Association's headquarters *55 Eton Avenue, London NW3 3ET*.

There is a cassette library for blind gardeners. The library contains recordings of handbooks issued by the Royal Horticultural Society and others, as well as extracts from weekly and monthly gardening journals. The library does not loan cassettes. Members have to send in their own cassettes in order to get copies of the master tapes held in the library. The one exception to this is the quarterly journal, *The Gardener*, which it is planned to publish again as from April 1982. The annual subscription of £1 to the Library will also provide members with quarterly copies of the magazine on cassette or in braille. On receipt of a subscription, the honorary librarian, Miss Kathleen Fleet, will supply posting instructions and a full list of the recordings available. Miss Fleet is also honorary information officer with the Advisory Committee for Blind Gardeners, which meets under the auspices of the Southern and Western Regional Association for the Blind. Having for many years also edited a gardening journal for the visually handicapped she is an invaluable source of information on all aspects of gardening, whether on methods suitable for a totally blind person or tools that are helpful to someone with very limited vision. Miss Fleet has written a book *Gardening without Sight* which will be published by the RNIB in print and braille towards the end of 1981. All enquiries and subscriptions (but no cassettes) should be sent to *Miss Kathleen Fleet, 48 Tolcarne Drive, Pinner, Middlesex HA5 2DQ (tel. 01-868 4026)*.

Handicrafts

People interested in handicrafts should be able to get help in developing their skills from the local authority or the local voluntary society, one or other of which in most areas will run craft groups especially for blind and handicapped people. It should also be possible with the help of the locally responsible society to get help in buying material cheaply, sometimes at a discount, often at trade rates. Basket-making still remains a satisfying skill, and visually handicapped people have successfully taken up a wide variety of hobbies including lampshade making, mosaic work, jewellery making, weaving, pottery and carpentry. To find out what is available in any given area, contact a local social worker.

A booklet *Woodwork for the Visually Handicapped*, written by Peter Jones, BEM, who is a blind 'do-it-yourself' enthusiast, is available from the RNIB. The print version is free, the braille edition costs 36p (concession price). The booklet lists a comprehensive range of woodworking tools generally available which are specially suitable for those with little or no sight. The booklet gives advice on making such items as a bookcase for braille books. Peter Jones is always glad to give advice on any specific woodwork problems. His address is *69 Prospect Road, Bradway, Sheffield S17 4JB (tel. Sheffield (0742) 36199)*.

Indoor games

A variety of games such as draughts, beetle, dominoes, backgammon, solitaire, are available from the RNIB with modifications to the usual designs to enable blind players to distinguish individual pieces, but all made so that both blind and sighted players can use them. There is even a small board for noughts and crosses marked out with nine holes into which either flat-ended or pointed pegs are put to represent the symbols. None of these adaptations require any knowledge of braille; on the dominoes for example, the pips are raised so that they can easily be felt; white draughtsmen are smaller than the black to make for easy distinction and the black squares on the board are slightly sunk. A wooden domino holder, designed by a blind man, John Broughton of Lincoln, is also available free from the RNIB.

The RNIB stocks a number of board games which use a colour coding system devised by another blind man, John Slade, in which different shapes indicate different colours. The games include Ludo and Hexehop (which is based on Chinese Chequers). Extra large dominoes which are also designed for visually-handicapped players, and extra large dice with very clear markings, can be obtained from *ESA Creative Learning Ltd, Fairview Road, Stevenage, Hertfordshire (tel. Stevenage (0438) 726383)*.

Extra large tactile dice are also available from the RNIB in half-inch cubes and ⅞-inch cubes. The RNIB sells a Scrabble set with a revolving board and alphabet tiles embossed in braille and inkprint.

186

People whose touch is poor often find that they can feel the very distinct dots on these tiles, but to play Scrabble effectively demands a good knowledge of the braille alphabet and a good memory. The RNIB also sells a set of Mastermind for the blind and has two different crossword puzzles which can be used by people with a good knowledge of braille. For more details of games suitable for blind children see Chapter 16, 'Parents and Children', pages 216–219.

Kate Shelley, who is blind, and her husband Dave, are enthusiastic players of board games; they have devised various ways of adapting the games to enable blind people to take part, with or without sighted players. Cards can be brailled, boards can be marked with dymo tape, or charted separately on a sheet of braille paper with numbers referring to the different sections of the board. Those who share their interest are invited to get in touch with them at *6 Buckingham Way, Wallington, Surrey SM6 9LT (tel. 01-647 3080)*.

Museums

While the museums in this country have not yet mounted a permanent exhibition designed for the blind, such as was opened at the Museum of Arts and History in Brussels in 1976, there has been a growing awareness by museums and art galleries of the special needs of visually handicapped people. The Museums Association regularly compiles a list of museums and galleries which provide special facilities for the blind. To get the free list send a stamped addressed envelope to the *Information Officer of the Museums Association, 34 Bloomsbury Way, London WC1 (tel. 01-404 4767)*.

An organisation called 'Art to Share' was set up in 1979 by Dr Sheila Smith of Nottingham University; she wanted to provide opportunities for blind and sighted people to compare their tactile and visual experiences of the arts. The organisation's first venture was a sculpture exhibition at the Nottingham Castle Museum where a number of discussion groups were held with the participation of the artists whose work was on view. 'Art to Share' is at the moment based in Nottingham, but it is hoped that it will grow into a national organisation. Enquiries to *Dr Smith, Senior Lecturer in English, University of Nottingham, University Park, Nottingham NG7 2RD*.

Music

Given a fluent knowledge of Grade 2 standard English braille, it is not too difficult to learn braille music. A recommended book for learning braille music is *Elementary Lessons and Exercises in Braille Music Notation* by Watson, available both in braille and inkprint from the RNIB. The RNIB has a large music department. The latest catalogue has about 5,000 titles ranging from classical to pop. New music publications are announced in *New Beacon* and in *Braille Monthly Announcements*. The RNIB also publishes *Braille Musical Magazine* monthly with articles of interest to both the amateur and the professional musician.

Braille music is sold at a discount to blind people ordinarily resident in the United Kingdom, but all the music in the RNIB's Braille Music Catalogue can be borrowed through the National Library for the Blind.

Transcribing music into braille
In theory, any music can be transcribed into braille, but in practice it is of doubtful value to transcribe vast orchestral scores because the finger cannot scan over several lines as an eye can. Standard braille music is now written 'bar over bar' that is, for a keyboard instrument, several bars of right-hand are printed consecutively along one line with the corresponding bars of left-hand below them. The old method 'bar by bar' (one left hand followed by one right hand) is not produced any more, though there is still a lot available from old stock. Most people find it quite easy to switch from one method to the other. The RNIB can arrange for music to be transcribed, if it is not available in the catalogue, but it is a lengthy process.

Large print music
Many visually handicapped people find it too difficult to learn braille music, but quite a few who have residual vision could read large print music, if it were available. However the provision is at the moment not very adequate. The majority of large print music produced in this country is aimed at children and is not likely to serve the needs of an adult musician who has begun to suffer from failing vision.

The only way in which large print music can be obtained is by having it specially copied on to large-sized music manuscript paper – or to have standard music photographically enlarged. The Partially Sighted Society's enlarging service was set up, partly to meet this need (for details of this service see page 72) but it may also be possible to get free enlargements for partially-sighted musicians from a well-disposed firm of architects – or town planners – who have suitable equipment. Following a request from *In Touch* a London firm undertook to do photographic enlargements of sheet music for a partially-sighted music teacher, and have expressed their willingness to do more. Contact *Seifert and Partners, 164 Shaftesbury Avenue, London WC2*.

In 1981, The Disabled Living Foundation published a resource paper on 'Music for the partially sighted' written by their music adviser, Daphne Kennard; this lists all known sources of help and gives information about various experiments with new aids in progress. The report is available free (in large print if required) from the DLF.

Opportunities for singers

Blind singers often join sighted choirs if they are expert at reading braille music. There are also a number of choirs for visually handicapped singers. In London the Pro Canto singers rehearse each week at the RNIB. Details from their conductor, *Peter Bamber, 19 Braemar Avenue, London N22 4BY (tel. 01-888 6271)*.

There is a long established choir in Leeds; for details contact *Mr H. Clarke, Social Services Department, Merrion House, 110 Merrion Centre, Leeds LS2 8QA (tel. (0532) 463411*. Another active group is the Dorset Blind Choir. Contact *Mrs H.M. Millett, 11 Highland Road, Parkstone, Poole, Dorset BH14 0DX (tel. Parkstone (0202) 744631)*.

Concessions for blind musicians

Under the terms of a legacy the RNIB has free tickets for most Royal Albert Hall concerts. These are given to blind musicians, though occasionally, if the tickets are not required by professionals, they can be issued to other blind music-lovers. Details from the RNIB's music department. The music department also has a panel of sighted professional musicians who will on request tape record music for blind colleagues. This service is only available for professional musicians.

Photography

A number of visually-handicapped people have found that enlarged photographs can help them to see objects which would otherwise be nearly invisible to them. Some are themselves very successful amateur photographers. Mr Bill Guard MBE, of Manchester, is not only a skilled photographer, but has also devised a way of making his own enlargements so that he can examine in detail the pictures he has taken of flowers, animals and landscapes. Even though he is now no longer taking photographs, he would still be glad to explain to others how he adapted his photographic equipment. His address is *33 Kingsholme Road, Manchester M22 6AQ (tel. Manchester (061) 437 2469)*.

Photography for the Disabled is a registered charity set up by amateur photographers who take a special interest in the problems of disabled people wanting to take up photography. Their president, Arthur Scrase, says that they will also be happy to try and help any visually handicapped people with the choice of equipment and put them in touch with local amateur photographers clubs where they might also get helpful advice. Contact him at *190 Secrett House, Ham Close, Ham, Richmond, Surrey TW10 7PE (tel. 01-948 2342)*.

Racing

A group of blind people led by Mrs Valerie Freedman, the wife of a well-known owner and breeder, organises regular trips to race meetings throughout the year. Mrs Freedman is also often able to arrange for members of the group to meet trainers, jockeys and other racing personalities. The number of people who can go to any particular race meeting has to be limited, and those living outside the London area must be prepared to make their own travelling arrangements to the rendezvous point. Any blind person who would be interested in going on the rota to join a group visit should contact *Harold Smith, Blind Racegoers, 66 Guinness Trust, Kennington Park Road, London SE11 4JF* (please send stamped, addressed envelope).

It is also possible to get a tactile map of Aintree racecourse to help blind racing enthusiasts follow the Grand National. Copies from *Reg Hunter, 197a Sutton Street, Liverpool L13 7EQ*.

Rambling

Although there are a number of blind ramblers groups (details of which can be obtained from the Sports and Recreation Officer at the RNIB), it would probably be possible for a competent blind walker to join in local groups organised by the Ramblers Association. (It might be advisable for a blind walker to come with a sighted companion – at least on the first occasion). For details of nearest local group contact the *Ramblers Association, 1-5 Wandsworth Road, London SW8 2LJ (tel. 01-582 6878)*.

Groups of blind ramblers can get help in planning routes from officials of the Forestry Commission, who can also sometimes provide guides. Those interested in exploring their own part of the country should enquire about this sort of help from the local conservancy office – there are eleven of them in England, Wales and Scotland, and the addresses and telephone numbers can be obtained from *The Forestry Commission, 231 Corstorphine Road, Edinburgh EH12 7AT (tel. Edinburgh (031) 334 0303)*.

Wardens in National Parks can also help with outings in rural areas. Each National Park has its own information service, the addresses of which can be obtained from *The Countryside Commission, John Dower House, Crescent Place, Cheltenham, Gloucestershire GL50 3RA (tel. Cheltenham (0242) 21381)*.

There are a number of nature trails specially adapted for the blind: one is in North London at Trent Park, Enfield and there are also Tollcross and Linn Nature Trails, both at Strathclyde, Glasgow, as well as a small area in the Tintern Forest and the Garth Falls Walk in Gwydyr Forest.

Sports

Many visually handicapped people contact local sports groups and find relatively little difficulty in joining in, provided the instructors are sympathetic to their problems. There are also throughout the country a number of sports clubs catering for the blind; full up-to-date details can be obtained from BASRAB or from the Sports and Recreations Officer of the RNIB.

In addition to sports listed separately in this chapter, many blind people are active in athletics, archery, horse-riding, judo, ski-ing, swimming and yachting.

Tandem cycling

Many blind people enjoy cycling, riding tandem with a sighted person. There are some local groups specifically for blind tandem enthusiasts. The Tandem Club has members all over Britain and would be willing to try to put a blind person in touch with a sighted tandem enthusiast in his own area. The Club has appointed Sue Atkin as its Liaison Officer for the Visually Handicapped. Mrs Atkin, who is blind, estimates that she and her husband cover about 7,000 miles a year on their tandem. She can be contacted at *15 Boundary House, St Margaret's Road, Twickenham TW1 1NW*.

The Cyclists Touring Club is also glad to try and help handicapped cyclists. Details of local district associations, some of which already have blind members, from the *Cyclists Touring Club, 69 Meadrow, Godalming, Surrey GU7 3HS (tel. Godalming (04868) 7217/9)*.

Both Clubs have journals containing information about tandems.

The British Cycling Bureau has a list of firms that hire tandems. Contact *Bicycle Association, Starley House, Eaton Road, Coventry CV1 2FH (tel. Coventry (0203) 27427)*.

The Peak District National Park hires tandems to disabled people. More details from the *Park Office, Aldern House, Baslow Road, Bakewell, Derbyshire (tel. 062 981 4321)*.

The Partially-Sighted Society has a tandem section run by *Mr Pat Smith, Anchor Garage and Cycles, Winchcombe, Gloucestershire GL54 5EE (tel. (0242) 602 550)*.

New tandems are expensive to buy, but it is sometimes possible to get a discount for a visually handicapped customer. A 15 per cent discount is offered by *The Tandem Centre, 281 Old Kent Road, London SE1 5JL (tel. 01-231 1641)*.

★   *Keep a simple length of string two yards long with knots a foot apart handy in the pocket. It is handy for all sorts of measuring jobs in house and garden. (Albert Wright, Farnham)*

★   *Use a child's bead frame to help remember how many rows you have knitted. Clip a small clothes peg between the beads, and move it along one bead after a row has been completed. (Gladys Archibald, Swalecliff)*

Travel and holidays

Cars and the Orange Badge scheme

To travel by car is probably the easiest method of transport for a blind person. Certain parking concessions are available to blind people under the Orange Badge scheme.

The Orange Badge, to be displayed in the windscreen, entitles the holder or his/her driver to park at meter bays without charge or time limit and for any length of time in streets where waiting is otherwise limited. Additionally, in England, Wales and Northern Ireland, badge holders may park their vehicles for up to two hours on single or double yellow lines except where a ban on loading and unloading is in force or in a bus lane. When parking on yellow lines a special parking disc must be displayed (in addition to the windscreen badge) which should be set to show time of arrival. In Scotland there is no limit for parking on yellow lines and the parking discs are not required.

Registered blind people are eligible for a Disabled Person's Badge which may be displayed in any vehicle in which the holder travels. In addition an Institution Badge is available to organisations concerned with the care of disabled people entitled to the concessions. This badge is intended for use in larger passenger vehicles, such as mini-buses, carrying groups of these disabled people.

The Orange Badge is valid for three years and must be renewed after that period. In England, Scotland and Wales applications should be made to the local social services department. In Northern Ireland applications should be sent to the nearest Roads Service Division of the Department of the Environment. In some parts of the country a fee is charged for the badge to cover administrative expenses. If the badge is no longer required by its holder it must be surrendered to the issuing authority. It must not be transferred to another person. It is also an offence for ineligible drivers to use the parking concessions bestowed by the badge if they are not transporting the badge holder at the time; and badge holders may risk forfeiting their badge if they allow their badges to be misused in this way. It is, therefore, advisable for badge holders to remove their badge from the vehicle when they are not travelling in it.

The holder's name is written on the badge and a vehicle registration number is required by law for local authority records, although the badge may be displayed in any vehicle in which the holder travels.

Also available, though not obligatory, are three different types of badge for display at the rear of vehicles so that those used by disabled or blind people will be easily recognised by other motorists.

The Orange Badge scheme applies throughout the United Kingdom with the exception of central London (the City of London, City of Westminster, the Royal Borough of Kensington and Chelsea and part of the London Borough of Camden). These boroughs operate their own concessionary schemes for blind people resident or working in the borough and also issue Orange Badges for use elsewhere, but the concessions bestowed by these are not available in the Inner London areas.

Until December 1975 when the Invalid Vehicles Scheme came to an end, an ordinary car was issued by the Department of Health and Social Security to a couple where one was registered blind and the other so handicapped as to be eligible for a Ministry invalid car. No more cars are now being issued to couples who have come into this category since 1 January 1976 when the Mobility Allowance was introduced – instead the disabled partner will get a Mobility Allowance (blind people who have no other handicaps do not qualify). But couples who had received a car while the scheme was in force are being allowed to keep it, and will have it replaced as long as they remain eligible under the rules of the old scheme.

Public transport
In Northern Ireland all registered blind people, regardless of age, can travel free on all buses and trains; unfortunately this general concession does not exist elsewhere in Britain. Instead there is a rather confusing variety of concessions applying to buses and underground trains, though towards the end of 1981 British Rail introduced (for a trial period) a Disabled Person's Railcard – for which registered blind and partially sighted people would be eligible. Blind people living in rural areas are obviously particularly affected by the decline of public transport in the countryside and are increasingly dependent on the goodwill of friends and relatives with cars. In addition to the concessions listed below, it is always worth checking with the local social services department or voluntary association about arrangements in their district: in some areas people are trying to arrange community bus services or car rotas to meet local needs. In one area a blind lady helps to co-ordinate the local drivers' scheme.

Bus travel
Many areas do have fare concessions for blind people, but the arrangements vary greatly. In some places the bus company or the local authority issues a special bus pass which enables a blind person to travel free; in some areas a single fare will cover both the blind person and guide. Often a concession scheme is advertised as being for pensioners who can travel at reduced fare outside the rush hours, but on enquiry it may be found that this scheme is intended also to apply to blind people irrespective of age. Elsewhere there may be no travel concessions at all. There are no fare concessions on long-distance coaches.

Stopping a bus (or taxi): The RNIB sells a bus card which can be held up by blind people at bus stops to show the number of the bus for which they are waiting. The cards consist of a ferrous metal plate welded into a black plastic wallet on to which white numbers three inches high made in magnetised rubber can be stuck. The card comes in two sizes; the smaller one (four inches by five inches) will take two digits and costs 89p (concession price); and the larger one (four inches by seven inches) will take three digits and costs £1.12 (concession price). The card design was suggested by a Londoner, Mr Joel Antrich; his wife Freda is nearly blind and had experienced great difficulties at request bus stops and those which served several different routes.

Mr Antrich was also responsible for the original design of the taxi card issued free by the RNIB. This is a plastic card, about the size of a £1 note, which has the word 'TAXI' printed boldly on both sides. Blind people who have used these cards report that taxi drivers are very appreciative of them as they are very easy to see.

British Rail
In 1981, British Rail announced a new travel concession in the form of a Disabled Person's Railcard. This costs £10 a year and enables half-price travel for the holder and a guide on all ordinary first and second class trips, and away-day fares – but not on other concessionary fares or season tickets. All registered blind and partially sighted persons will be eligible for a Disabled Person's Railcard – but they must be able to produce proof of registration, which need not be a specially prepared document. Any document, such as that used to obtain previous travel concessions or the reduced TV licence would be

acceptable. Those who do not have such a document would need to request it from the local authority where they are registered. The British Rail scheme is being introduced for a trial period initially and will be reassessed at the end of 1982. British Rail state that they are prepared to make arrangements to help any disabled passengers have as comfortable a journey as possible. Arrangements can be made to meet a passenger at the departure station, escort him or her safely on to the train, and similar arrangements can be made at the destination station or any intermediate changing point. In large cities, a disabled passenger can also be helped with interchange from one station to another. Blind people travelling alone who wish to take advantage of this service should give advance warning (at least one day) to the station master at the station where the journey begins. British Rail has also waived its rule against dogs in sleepers to allow guide dog owners to travel with ease. Blind travellers with guide dogs will be accommodated in first-class compartments, if space is available, but only charged the second-class fare. It is necessary to provide a vet's certificate stating that the guide dog is in good health. British Rail also now allows guide dogs to accompany their owners into restaurant cars and buffet cars.

Underground travel

There are only four underground systems in British cities, and as many variations in the concessions available to blind passengers! In Glasgow there are no special concessions for the blind, but all passengers pay a flat fare rate irrespective of whether they are travelling from one station to the next, or for the length of the line. In Liverpool all registered blind people can travel free – at all times – on the underground and the Merseyrail service provided they have a travel pass issued by the social services department. In Newcastle all employed blind people are eligible for free travel at all times; all other blind people can get free travel at off-peak times. In London there are travel concessions available only to working blind people who can, on production of a pass issued by the local social services department, travel anywhere on the London underground at any time for 20p. But blind people who continue to work after retirement age may then be restricted to the off-peak concessionary fares available to all other elderly people.

Long-distance travel
Concessions are available to a blind person accompanied by a guide on inland flights by domestic airlines in the United Kingdom. If the journey is in connection with work or training for employment, or in connection with medical treatment or rehabilitation the blind traveller or the local authority can apply to the airline for a certificate, which has to be signed by a blind welfare authority and then presented when buying the air ticket. The blind traveller and guide in these circumstances can travel on payment of one full fare. No concessions are given at present by any airlines for travel outside the United Kingdom. Travelling by sea is a little easier, however. All shipping lines of the North Atlantic Shipping Conference (which covers most British shipping lines on the transatlantic crossing) accept a blind person's guide at half the regular fare, if the blind person is travelling in the course of business or professionally. Applications for this concession must be backed by a letter from the RNIB.

Inquiries about travel concessions abroad should be made to the appropriate organisation for the blind in that country. A list of such organisations appears in the RNIB's Directory of Agencies.

Escorts
Finding an escort is often a problem for a blind person who is unused to travelling, or needs to make a journey on an unfamiliar route. Both the Red Cross and the WRVS can usually help here, if contacted in good time. They would be prepared to help take someone to hospital, or to a rehabilitation centre, or escort a child to residential school and might also consider 'social' journeys (a visit to relatives, for instance) if there is no more urgent call on their helpers' time. Applications should be made to the nearest branch; the address should be obtainable from the local post office. Blind people travelling by train, coach or air, who arrive at one London terminus and have to cross the city to another should contact the Southern and Western Regional Association for the Blind. This association can arrange for someone, generally a member of the Red Cross, to escort blind travellers across London, and help them safely on to the next stage of their journey. Again, it is necessary to give advance warning of travel plans.

Holiday hotels for the blind

There are fifteen hotels specially catering for the needs of blind and partially sighted holiday makers in England and Wales. The hotels are all run by voluntary societies for the blind: four of them by the Royal National Institute for the Blind, the others by various local voluntary societies. There are no special hotels in Scotland or Northern Ireland but all the hotels will take registered blind and partially sighted guests from all parts of Britain.

The hotels will accept bookings from visually handicapped people who are also deaf, but they require them to be accompanied by a sighted companion. The hotels will also welcome a sighted relative or friend accompanying a blind guest, and many of them will also accept the sighted children of blind parents.

Almost all the hotels will provide special diets (for diabetics, for instance) and with advance notice the management can arrange for a district nurse to give injections or administer eye drops for a blind holidaymaker. But the hotels are not in a position to cope with guests who are not in reasonable health. Most managers say that they will accept unaccompanied blind people as guests, provided that they are independent and capable of looking after themselves. But although some hotels have arrangements with local volunteers to act as escorts for blind visitors, the managers have pointed out that a blind person in an unfamiliar environment is more likely to enjoy a holiday if accompanied by a sighted guide.

None of the hotels listed below is purpose built to meet the needs of blind people, but they all claim to have guide rails, stair guards, grab-rails in baths and so on, to help avoid hazards which might worry elderly blind holidaymakers. Most hotels have lifts, and the list below indicates where ground floor accommodation is available in those hotels without lifts. All hotels (except the Chaucer House, Skegness) will accept guide dogs, but some may not permit them in the dining-room.

Details of the hotels including weekly charges (correct for 1981 holiday season) and numbers of rooms are given below. Unless otherwise stated, enquiries can be made direct to the hotel, and blind people who are going to pay for their holiday themselves need not apply through a social worker. Bookings usually start immediately after Christmas for the summer season, and it is advisable to book as early as possible.

Hotels usually ask for a small deposit on booking, and full payment is required to be made about three or four weeks in advance of the booking. Advance payment is requested because vacancies arising from last-minute cancellations are difficult to fill at short notice, and the hotels, which are heavily subsidised from voluntary funds, are anxious to minimise costs. But if holidaymakers have to cancel for unavoidable reasons, such as illness, the hotels would give sympathetic consideration to requests for refunds.

Most holiday hotels for the blind are open only during the holiday season, but many residential homes for the blind are prepared to take short-term guests at any time of the year, if they have a vacancy. Weekly charges are higher than for holiday hotels, but permanent homes are usually better equipped to accommodate the elderly and frail who need more care and attention. A complete list of homes for the blind in England and Wales can be obtained free from the RNIB. Those who need temporary accommodation during the absence of relatives, for example, but who are too frail to travel any distance, may find that the local authority can offer a place in one of its own old people's homes.

The Torch Trust for the Blind can offer short-stay accommodation to a very limited number of people who wish to have Christian Fellowship while on holiday. Neither Torch House, at Hallaton in Leicestershire, nor the Trust's other property, 'Little Torch' at Hurstpierpoint in Sussex, are hotels; but the directors, Ron and Stella Heath, are very sympathetic to those who need rest and refreshment as well as an understanding listener with whom to discuss problems.

Addresses and details

Abergele, Clwyd: Llys Onnen Home for the Blind
Open all year round; £55 per week.
5 single, 5 twin-bedded, 5 family rooms; no lift, but some accommodation on the ground floor.
Applications to: North Wales Society for the Blind, 325 High Street, Bangor, Gwynedd LL57 1YB (tel. Bangor (0248) 53604).

Blackpool, Lancashire: Century Hotel (RNIB)
£42 per week for June/July/August, £38 per week during low season, £47 per week at Christmas.
4 single, 6 double, 17 twin-bedded rooms.
Address: 406 North Promenade, Gynn Square, Blackpool FY1 2LB (tel. Blackpool (0253) 54598).

Blackpool, Lancashire: Henderson Holiday Home for the Blind
Open from Easter to mid-October; £36 per week; no special diets catered for; only one guide dog accepted at a time.
10 single, 3 double, 12 twin-bedded rooms.
Address: 1 Wimborne Place, South Shore, Blackpool.
Applications to: Liverpool Voluntary Society for the Blind, 18 Slater Street, Liverpool L1 4BS (tel. 051-709 2398).

Bognor Regis, Sussex: Russell Hotel
Open from mid-April to end October, also Christmas; £45 per week.
Run by London Association for the Blind; apply direct (see address below).
10 single, 16 double rooms.
Address: King's Parade, Bognor Regis, Sussex PO21 2QP (tel. Bognor Regis (0243) 823572).

Eastbourne, Sussex: Palm Court Hotel (RNIB)
Open from Easter to end October, also Christmas; £42 per week for June/July/August, £38 per week during low season, £47 per week at Christmas.
13 single, 19 twin-bedded, 2 three-bedded rooms.
Address: 15 Burlington Place, Eastbourne, Sussex BN21 4AR (tel. Eastbourne (0323) 25811).

Felixstowe, Suffolk: Savile Court
Open from April to October; £60 for 11 days *or* if guest is from area covered by East Suffolk Association for the Blind £27.50 for 11 days.
1 single, 6 double, 1 three-bedded rooms; no lift, but some accommodation on the ground floor.
Applications to: East Suffolk Association for the Blind, County Buildings, Cumberland Street, Woodbridge, Suffolk (tel. Woodbridge (03943) 4161).

Llandudno, Gwynedd (North Wales): Belmont Hotel
Open from Easter to November, also two weeks at Christmas; £40 per week.
7 single, 1 double, 2 family, 18 twin-bedded rooms, all but 4 accessible by lift.
Applications to: Henshaws Society for the Blind, Warwick Road, Old Trafford, Manchester M16 0GS (tel. 061-872 1234/5).

Llandudno, Gwynedd (North Wales): Howard Hotel (RNIB)
Open from Easter to end October, also Christmas; £42 per week for
June/July/August, £38 per week during low season, £47 per week at
Christmas.
7 single, 16 double- or two-/three-bedded rooms.
Address: Gloddaeth Crescent, Central Promenade, Llandudno,
Gwynedd LL30 2XT (tel. Llandudno (0492) 77770).

Margate, Kent: Merrell House
Open from April to October; £34 per week *or* if guest is from area
covered by Kent Association for the Blind £28 per week for period
June/July/August; rates reduced outside this main holiday season;
sighted children not accepted.
4 two-bedded, 3 three-bedded rooms; no lift, but 2 bedrooms on
ground floor.
Applications to: Kent Association for the Blind, 15 Ashford Road,
Maidstone, Kent (tel. Maidstone (0622) 58717/54448).

Morecambe, Lancashire: Welson Holiday Hotel for the Blind
Open from Easter to October, also 1 week at Christmas; £50 per week
plus VAT from 30 May–29 August, rates reduced outside this main
holiday season.
4 single, 9 double, 11 twin-bedded rooms; 4 rooms in basement not
accessible by lift.
Applications to: Institute for Blind Welfare, Lytham Road, Fulwood,
Preston, Lancashire (tel. Preston (0772) 717295/6).

Scarborough, North Yorkshire: Alma Court Hotel (RNIB)
Open from Easter to mid-October, also Christmas; £42 per week for
June/July/August, £38 per week during low season, £47 per week at
Christmas.
18 single, 10 double, 3 family bedrooms.
Address: West Street, Scarborough, North Yorkshire (tel. Scar-
borough (0723) 72934).

Skegness, Lincolnshire: Chaucer House
Open mid-May to end September, also Christmas; £35 per week;
children and guide dogs not accepted.
Applications to: Royal Midland Institute for the Blind, Chaucer Street,
Nottingham NG1 5LR (tel. Nottingham (0602) 42536).

Weston-super-Mare, Avon: Lauriston Hotel
Open 25 April to 14 November, also Christmas; £44 per week June to mid-September, £36 per week other times; reduction for children; 10-day booking also accepted. Run by London Association for the Blind; apply direct (see address below).
10 single, 15 double rooms.
Address: 6-8 Knightstone Road, Weston-super-Mare, Avon BS23 2AN (tel. Weston-super-Mare (0934) 20758).

Hotels for blind people with additional disabilities

Burnham-on-Sea, Somerset: Kathleen Chambers Home for the Deaf-Blind (RNIB)
Residential home for elderly deaf-blind (maximum accommodation 36 people) also accepts short-term guests for holidays or breaks; £42 per week for June/July/August, £38 per week during low season, £47 per week at Christmas. Only one guide dog accepted at a time. Children not accepted, so not suitable for families; but provides a secure environment for elderly people who simply wish to rest and be taken care of. There is a large garden, where they can walk safely. The home has no bar, and is a mile away from the town, so only likely to appeal to those more active guests who want a very quiet holiday and like walking; the beach is half a mile away across dunes.
No lift, but most rooms are on ground floor.
Address: 97 Berrow Road, Burnham-on-Sea, Somerset (tel. Burnham-on-Sea (0278) 782142).

Clacton-on-Sea, Essex: St Anne's Holiday Home for the Blind-Deaf
Open all year round; £50 per week from 10 June to 8 September; £42 per week from 15 April to 10 June, and from 9 September to 31 October, Christmas week £60; at all other times £32 per week; discretionary reduction in rates for guides who are not members of the family. Not suitable for children unless part of a family.
Accommodation for 14 guests, mainly in twin-bedded rooms; 2 rooms on ground floor for those who cannot manage stairs.
Address: 26-8 Harold Road, Clacton-on-Sea, Essex (tel. Clacton-on-Sea (0255) 20595).

Helston, Cornwall: Mill View Home for the Handicapped
Open from April to September; between £48 and £68 per week
according to season; reduced charges for children under 11, no charge
for toddlers. Caters for people with all kinds of disabilities, including
incontinence; will accept bookings only from groups of handicapped
people – though these do not have to be organised by official Institutions or Homes. Groups must number at least 12, not more than 21, in
main holiday season; but at other times smaller groups can be considered.
Address: Ruan Minor, Helston, Cornwall (tel. The Lizard (032 629)
0467).

Diabetics
Details of hotels which provide special diets for diabetics can be
obtained from the British Diabetic Association, 10 Queen Anne
Street, London W1M 0BD (tel. 01-323 1531).

Self-catering holidays

Hove, Sussex: Wavertree House
One of the RNIB's residential homes, this offers some bed and
breakfast accommodation at £20 per person per week. There is also a
self-contained fully furnished and equipped family flat for self-
catering holiday guests. This has a double bedroom and a twin-
bedded room and costs £65 per week.
Enquiries: RNIB Homes Department, 224 Great Portland St, London
W1N 6AA (tel. 01-388 1266).

St Leonards-on-Sea, West Sussex
The Middlesex Association for the Blind has two six-berth caravans
here, which are let at a subsidised rental (£40 per week) to registered
blind and partially sighted people and their families.
Enquiries: 83 Cambridge Street, London SW1V 4PG (tel. 01-828
8250).

Strathyre, West Perth (Scotland): Sir Andrew Murray House
Four self-catering suites are available for holiday use by blind and
partially sighted people and their families. Each suite consists of a
large bedroom, with cooking facilities; there is a separate kitchen and

dining room also available for any party of holidaymakers which occupies all four suites. The cost is £20 per suite per week, plus heating and lighting.

Enquiries: Mr P. Dukes, Central Regional Council, Social Work Department, Llarggarth, Viewforth, Stirling FK8 2ET (tel. Stirling (0786) 3111).

Help with the cost of holidays
In previous years local authorities were often able to help blind people in need with the cost of a holiday. But this may not always now be possible because of expenditure cuts. However a blind person in special need of a holiday, particularly if recovering from illness or after a bereavement, should make contact with their local social worker to see if they can help. Visually handicapped people who cannot afford to go on holiday independently might find that their local voluntary society for the blind can help, even if it does not have its own hotel or run a group holiday. Local voluntary societies are nearly always willing to contribute something towards the expense of a holiday, or will even meet the full cost in case of read need. Other charities such as Rotary and Lions may also be able to help. Some Rotary Clubs run group holidays – the address of the District Secretary can be obtained if necessary from *Rotary International, Sheen Lane House, Sheen Lane, London SW14 8AF (tel. 01-878 0931)*.

The Lions Clubs may also be able to provide financial help; they have their own holiday home for the blind at Great Yarmouth, which has room for about 25 people. Blind visitors need to be able to climb stairs, as there is no lift, and to be in reasonably good health as staff are unable to provide much in the way of medical attention. Accommodation is mainly in twin-bedded rooms. Blind guests and their guides are sponsored by local Lions Clubs, who are responsible for making all the arrangements, including travel, and pay the whole cost. Addresses of local Lions Clubs can be obtained from *Lions International Secretariat, 22 Craddock Street, Swansea, West Glamorganshire SA1 3HE (tel. Swansea (0792) 461305)*.

More active holidaymakers may be able to obtain financial help from a charity linked to the Countrywide Holidays Association, for holidays at any of the guest houses it has in many different parts of Britain. The cost at one of these centres varies between £60 and £90 a week, and the Association arranges holidays with day walking excursions, or catering for special interests such as painting, photography, music or dancing. It cannot provide guides for blind visitors, but will arrange holidays for blind individuals, or for groups, if required. Further information from the *Countrywide Holidays Association, Birch Heys, Cromwell Range, Manchester M14 6HU (tel. 061-224 2887)*.

In recent years, increasing numbers of voluntary societies and local authorities have arranged group holidays for blind, partially-sighted and physically handicapped people. Generally a hotel or boarding house is taken over by a party for a week or a fortnight, either early or late in the holiday season. Transport is provided and entertainments and outings arranged. This can be a very friendly, happy holiday, and a good way for a person whose sight has only recently deteriorated to take the first big step of leaving known surroundings and yet have the support of friends made amongst blind people in the locality. Saga, a tour operator which specialises in holidays for people over retiring age, is hoping to arrange more holidays for the disabled, including the visually handicapped, and would welcome enquiries. Contact *Paul Bach, Marketing Manager, Saga Travel Service, PO Box 64, 119 Sandgate Road, Folkestone, Kent CT20 2BN (tel. Folkestone (0303) 30000)*.

In recent years a number of holidays have been organised to give blind people a chance to try activities ranging from sailing to pony-trekking. In some areas these have been arranged by local voluntary associations and in other places an enterprising mobility officer has been the organiser. It should be possible to get details of schemes which are not purely local from the Sports and Recreation Officer of the RNIB.

Many other activities centres welcome individuals with a visual or other handicap. Some may consider arranging special courses if approached by a group of blind people. The Central Bureau for Educational Visits and Exchanges has information about a wide variety of sporting and educational activities taking place in this country, and will gladly help visually handicapped holidaymakers from this country as well as from abroad. One particularly useful brochure which can be obtained from the Central Bureau is called 'Young Visitors to Britain'. It contains details of all kinds of adventurous holidays. Those which can accommodate blind or other disabled youngsters are indicated.. Contact the *Central Bureau for Educational Visits and Exchanges, 43 Dorset Street, London W1H 3FN (tel. 01-486 5101)*.

Group holidays have not been restricted to resorts in Britain. Several have ventured abroad. One of the pioneers was the Chichester Adventure Club, which was organised by local blind people.

For the last few years, group holidays to Spain have been arranged (and Kathy Page, the organiser, takes pride in the fact that the party has included several people over 80!) by the *Royal Sheffield Institution for the Blind, 5 Mappin Street, West Street, Sheffield, South Yorkshire S1 4DT (tel. Sheffield (0742) 22757)*.

In 1980, the Hampshire Association for the Blind (which has always organised a number of activity holidays in its own area) took a group of blind holiday-makers abroad in a group jointly organised with the Leicestershire Society for the Blind. Contact *Hampshire Association for the Care of the Blind, 4 Southgate Street, Winchester, Hampshire SO23 9EF (tel. Winchester (0962) 65570)* or *Royal Leicestershire, Rutland and Wycliffe Society for the Blind, Margaret Road, Leicester, Leicestershire LE5 5FU (tel. Leicester (0533) 736562)* for details of future holiday plans.

Independent holidays

Several helpful books are available for those who do not wish to have a holiday in a group but feel they need some extra help in choosing a suitable holiday spot. The Royal Association for Disability and Rehabilitation publish annually a substantial book entitled *Holidays for the Physically Handicapped* which is packed with useful information. Major resorts are briefly described, with special emphasis on how level or hilly they are. Hotels and boarding houses are listed with details of ground-floor accommodation, access to toilets, suitability for wheelchair users, closeness to shops or seafront, as well as their weekly charges. The book also includes information about the possibility of visitors bringing guide dogs. The AA also issues a *Guide for the Disabled* which gives similar details about AA recommended hotels, guest houses and farm houses. Guide dog owners can also get lists of suitable holiday camps and boarding houses from the Guide Dogs for the Blind Association. Helpful booklets about holiday possibilities are issued by the Chest and Heart Association, the Spastics Society and the British Diabetic Association.

Educational holidays

Arising out of a suggestion made on the *In Touch* programme, a special summer school for the blind was organised by the Association for Blind and Partially Sighted Teachers and Students at Leeds University in 1973. This proved so popular that similar schools have been held at Leeds and elsewhere every summer since then. The subjects studied have ranged from marine biology and industrial archaeology to music, drama and politics. No one organisation is responsible for all the various schools but ABAPSTAS is likely to be aware of what is being arranged. Write to the ABAPSTAS secretary for details.

Holidays abroad
Most holiday accommodation for blind people on the Continent tends to be fully booked by nationals of the host country. However, some organisations for the blind in European countries would be prepared to take holiday guests from other countries at their own holiday homes during off peak periods.

Italy
There is a hotel run by the local organisation of the blind at Tirrenia, a few miles from Pisa, and close to the sea. For full information contact *Unione Italiana dei Ciechi, Via Borgognona 38, 00187, Rome (tel. 68 92 02)*.

West Germany
There are hotels for blind holiday-makers on the North Sea coast, and in the mountains. Details from *Deutscher Blindenverband, Bismarck-allee 30, 5300 Bonn 2 (tel. 35 30 19)*.

Sweden
There are several hotels for the blind. Details from *Synskadades Riksforbund, 52 PA 122 88, Enskede Växel (tel. 39 00 20)*.

Luxembourg
In Luxembourg there is a purpose-built hotel, situated in a park with marked walks and a heated swimming pool. Details from *Home national de l'association des Aveugles du Luxembourg, 47 rue de Luxembourg, Bershbach/Mersch, Grand Duchy of Luxembourg*.

Switzerland
There are two hotels catering for blind visitors. One is in Saanen, a village 1150 metres above sea level, in the Bernese Oberland near Gstaad. Contact *Ferienheim Solsane, Saanen 3780*.

207

The other hotel is on Lake Constance in a village about 420 metres above sea level. Contact *Blindenzentrum St Gebhardshohe, Bahnstation Munsterlingen CH-8597 Landschlacht*.

Elsewhere it may always be worthwhile for blind travellers to contact the local organisations of the blind who may well be able to give advice about local facilities. The RNIB's Directory of Agencies for the Blind has a full list of organisations of and for the blind in all parts of the world.

International home exchange scheme
The National Federation of the Blind has been trying to set up a scheme whereby blind people and their families could spend holidays free of charge abroad in return for offering hospitality in Britain. Full details from *David Mann, 107 Richmond Road, Montpelier, Bristol 6 (tel. Bristol (0272) 421950)*.

★   *Finding your room when you are staying in a strange place can be difficult. To avoid the embarrassment of walking into the wrong bedroom, take a supply of brightly coloured luggage labels whenever you are away from home and tie one to the door handle of your bedroom. A large rubber-band twisted round the door knob will do the same for someone who is totally blind. (Dr Eleanor Sawdon, Croydon)*

★   *Always put a distinguishing mark on your luggage. Either attach a brightly-coloured label or something else which will enable you – or any helper – to pick it out from all the other similar suitcases and bags. I stick brightly-coloured strips of sticky paper across my case – and it is easy to spot a green case with red and yellow stripes! Obviously, if you have a little vision, be sure to pick a colour that you can see well yourself! (Jane Finnis)*

Parents and children

Visual handicap is a major problem for a tiny minority of children; only one child in every 6,000 is likely to be blind. Unfortunately, it is also true that for this minority of children visual handicap is unlikely to be their only handicap. Consequently, parents will be fortunate indeed if they have quick and easy access to professionals with first-hand knowledge of blind children, and it is unlikely that the first people parents turn to when they are seriously worried about their child's sight – the health visitor and family doctor – will have had any experience of severe visual handicap even when it is not masked or complicated by another handicap. There is, however, a great deal of help and advice available, both at professional and non-professional levels, if parents can bring themselves to seek it out. This chapter aims to point parents and professionals in the right direction to find the help they need, and to reassure the former that they do not have to be 'experts' to care tenderly, imaginatively and positively for their child.

Detecting visual handicap

Contrary to popular belief, defective sight in small children is not always obvious. Some parents have even found it difficult to convince professionals that their child has defective vision. It is hard to believe that the toddler who will happily sprawl on the garden path and follow the movements of an ant with a finger tip has a sight problem. It is only too easy to account for the fact that children constantly trip over steps, and bump into things, to their having been 'born clumsy' – and not to suspect that they have only a limited field of vision. A baby with very little sight may be such a 'very good' baby, lying contentedly in the pram, gazing upward with nothing obviously wrong and being no trouble to anyone. Simple tests which anyone can carry out at home include checking if the baby's eyes turn towards the ray of light from a torch (though it is vital to make sure no click is made as it is switched on, or the child will turn to that) or spinning a coin on the table. Here the trick is to watch what happens when the coin is silent. Is a hand reached out to try to grasp it? A few Smarties scattered on a light background can also give a mother a rough idea as to the kind of vision problem her child has; 'hundreds and thousands' can be used in the same way for a more difficult test.

Early diagnosis is essential if the child is to be helped to make the best use of any residual vision and parents should press for developmental tests at their clinic if they are seriously worried. Their GP can refer them to a children's development unit (paediatric assessment centre). Here a team of people, led by a paediatrician (a doctor specialising in the health of children) and including educational psychologists, physiotherapists and occupational therapists, will monitor the child's development. The best units will make the parents feel part of the assessment team, for only the parents can contribute intimate knowledge of the child based on almost continuous observation. Some units have playgroups attached, which the handicapped child can attend regularly. The assessment process should provide the basic information needed on which a programme of education and treatment can be based and also refer the parents to appropriate sources of help outside the unit.

It is only too likely that a child with more than one handicap will also be examined by other specialists, perhaps at different hospitals, according to the nature of these other disabilities and so that other health aspects can be checked out. With so many hospital appointments, parents may be forgiven for thinking that sometimes the left hand does not know what the right hand is doing, and that no one is prepared to give them a straight answer to anything. These anxieties are now being recognised, and it is recommended practice that one professional is designated as 'the named person' and his or her role is to act as a co-ordinator and as the first point of contact for parents in this situation.

When visual handicap is diagnosed, it is likely that the parents will be offered genetic counselling unless blindness is obviously due to environmental causes, such as rubella in pregnancy. Blindness in childhood is a complex subject, but it is generally held that genetic disorders are frequently responsible; so if counselling is not offered, parents should make certain it has not been mentioned because it was unnecessary, rather than because it had been overlooked.

Aids and equipment
Fortunately, visually handicapped children need little special equipment at home. Some items found in high street shops such as the chiming toothbrush and chiming hairbrush made by Tommee Tippee have been found to be popular, and have encouraged children to

persevere with unwelcome chores. An electric toothbrush with a large grip handle has appealed to others who hate cleaning their teeth. Stair safety gates can be obtained from Mothercare, as can bed rails for use on a divan bed. A musical potty has been found helpful in toilet training and can be obtained from Newton Aids who also issue a useful catalogue called 'Best Buys' which includes play tables, non-tip meal trays and a two handled three-quarter pint beaker. Contact *Newton Aids Ltd, Unit 4, Dolphin Industrial Estate, Southampton Road, Salisbury, Wiltshire (tel: Salisbury (0722) 20441).*

Play tables can also be made very successfully at home, as long as it is remembered that a raised lip around the edges is essential to stop things falling off.

Early days

All babies are special, but it is a rare parent who does not feel that a blind baby is 'extra special'. And indeed he is, though it is important to remember that first and foremost he is a *baby*. Because of not being able to see, more and different kinds of help are needed than for other babies, but the basic needs are just the same. In the first year, touch is the most important form of communication. Sighted children follow their mother's movements around the room with their eyes, but the blind baby will need her touch as the reassurance of her presence. Later, her voice will be connected to her presence, her footsteps will become meaningful and her scent will be comforting. But at first her distinctive way of holding the baby, her special tickle or caress are all important. Even so, if the baby has very little sight, there may seem to be no response. His face may seem distressingly blank to his mother if there is no eye-to-eye contact. Yet, although the baby's face does not light up, his movements in her arms will be quite different from those made when held by anyone else. When she speaks the baby may tend to be still in order to listen more attentively, and his hands will finger her face with an exploratory movement as if re-charting well-loved territory. Before the baby is ready to reach out to the intriguing noise made by a toy she holds, his or her fingers will start moving, sending the message 'I am interested' even if the face does not show it. The response is there, and by watching closely, the mother can learn this language and so cement the bond between the two of them.

As the baby grows, so also must the mother's ingenuity increase as she tries to show, in meaningful ways, all the hundred and one

211

everyday things sighted children absorb through their eyes. The task sounds daunting, but is one that should be shared by all the family, and brothers and sisters are often the most invaluable helpers.

Background reading
There are some excellent publications especially written to help families in this situation, though it is rather sad to note that most of them are American! For the busy parent, with little time to read, two small booklets entitled 'Get a Wiggle On' and 'Move It' aim to meet the needs of parents of blind children from birth to school age. They are attractively designed, and give a great deal of useful information crisply and cheerfully, yet in a way that catches the imagination and gives insight into the problems a blind child faces. The booklets can be obtained through the RNIB Education Department.

Can't Your Child See? (E.P. Scott, J.E. Jan and R.D. Freeman, University Park Press, 1977) is a much more substantial book, but again is very practical and realistic. It deals in detail with the child's early years, with a wealth of information as to ways of helping a blind child learn to stand and finally to walk, methods of encouraging language, coping with feeding problems and toilet training. It looks squarely at the problems of living with a visually handicapped child (one section is entitled 'When you feel like blowing your top') and discusses blind mannerisms frankly. One chapter concentrates on the needs of the multiply handicapped child. There is a wealth of first-hand anecdote which makes the book compulsive reading.

Children with a Severe Visual Defect (RNIB) is a useful British publication which has the additional merit of being free. It is written especially for mothers with children under three years of age, but mothers with older children who are slow in learning would also find it helpful.

The Psychoanalytic Study of the Child (Vol. 34, ed. A. Solmit, Yale University Press, 1979) contains two papers which would be especially useful for professionals – though parents should also find them of interest. These are *The Ordinary Devoted Mother and her Blind Baby*, by D.M. Wills, and *The Blind Nursery School Child*, by A. Curson. They are both based on research undertaken with blind children at the Hampstead Child-Therapy Course and Clinic.

Insights from the Blind (S. Fraiberg, Souvenir Press, 1977, £2.95) is a fascinating psychoanalytical study of a group of congenitally blind children which gives fresh insight into the perception and development of blind children.

Where to get help

However helpful books may be, contact with people who understand the problems and the anxieties that all parents of a handicapped child experience is often the most valuable help of all. There are a number of agencies outside the medical field to which parents can turn for advice and help. The quality of the help provided varies very much from area to area; it is unlikely that all the services mentioned here will be available in any one area. However, all the services have one thing in common: they aim to help parents care for their child in the security of its own home and to give practical help, advice and support throughout a very difficult period of the parents' marriage and family life. To ask for this help will not be interpreted as a request for the child 'to be put away'. This out-of-date phrase still rings down the years, and finds an echo in the anxious minds of mothers who may well be burdened with undisclosed fears about their handicapped child's future. Nowadays it is indeed a phrase of the past; services today are firmly home-based.

Social services departments

These have responsibilities for all visually handicapped children whether they are registered blind or partially sighted, or not yet registered as either (see page 21). A social worker will be able to advise on local sources of help and also provide, or give advice about, any aids or equipment that might be helpful. Aids can range from lifting equipment, such as hoists, to tiny items, such as suction egg cups or audible balls. Some social services departments have a counselling service for mothers of visually handicapped children, and provide opportunities for them to meet other parents for informal discussion and mutual support.

Local education authorities (LEAs)

Some LEAs now employ educational advisers, or peripatetic teachers for the visually handicapped, to give parents advice and guidance on education. An increasing number of these workers are trained and knowledgeable in child development and learning processes, and are able to offer expert help to mothers of pre-school children as well as to those with children of school age. Some peripatetic teachers for the visually handicapped are based at blind schools, others work from county council headquarters. Parents can find out whether this service exists in their area – and whether the service is appropriate to their needs – by discussing it with their social worker, found either at the hospital they attend or at their local social services department area office, or with their health visitor.

RNIB Education Advisory Service
This service brings practical and supportive help to the parents of young blind and partially sighted children. The ten education advisers – all of whom are professionally qualified, principally as teachers of the blind – function on a regional basis and their skills and experience bring support to parents, local authorities, and anyone concerned with the care and education of visually handicapped children. The service is not limited to pre-school children, but also offers practical advice and help in respect of visually handicapped children in normal schools, day special schools, hospitals, and any situation other than a school for the visually handicapped. The service is described in a free leaflet supplied by the RNIB, entitled *Education Advisory Services*, and can be contacted through the RNIB Education Department.

RNIB Telephone Advisory Service
This experimental twenty-four-hour service was set up in 1980 and any parent with a blind child, or any blind parent, can ring Mrs Gill Hinds. She is the wife of a RNIB education adviser and, although blind herself, is the mother of two children with normal sight. If parents wish it, she may be able to introduce them to other parents of blind children and she is a mine of up-to-date information or help available, and can give support and advice based both on her experience and that of many mothers with blind children. The telephone number is *Northampton (0604) 407726*.

The Partially Sighted Society
This society (see also page 24) has local branches and these may provide meeting places for parents whose children have eye defects but retain some useful vision. Where branches exist, they can give

214

support and encouragement to parents whose children have only recently been diagnosed as having very poor sight, and can give an invaluable consumer's guide to the facilities for such children in their locality. Information sheets on education and other publications are available from the Society and a Vice-President, George Marshall, OBE, has written a number of pamphlets on the needs and help available for partially sighted children. A full list of these publications can be obtained direct from *Mr Marshall, Waterside, The Green, Long Itchington, Rugby, Warwickshire*.

The National Association for Deaf-Blind and Rubella Handicapped

An association of parents, teachers and professionals concerned with all problems of deaf/blindness. The association has two centres (see page 255 and 256) which are open for holidays and emergency admissions, and four caravans in various parts of the country for holiday use. Meetings are held in various areas for parents of deaf-blind children and young people to discuss common problems, and a quarterly newsletter giving information on the progress of children is issued. Publications include *A Parent's Guide to the Early Care of a Deaf-Blind Child* by Peggy Freeman, a founder member of the Association and a *Progress Guide for Deaf-Blind and/or Severely Handicapped Children*. This guide, 'born out of the bewildered cry of many parents', aims to help them monitor their child's development, for with multiply-handicapped children development may be so slow that it is difficult to recognise that the child is, in fact, making progress, or to know what the next goal should be. A full list of the Association's publications and films is available on request.

Toy Library Association

This association is especially concerned that all handicapped children should have access to toys and activities that will help in their development. The association will put parents in touch with their nearest toy library and its advisory panel will answer specific queries from parents about play and handicap. Their Noah's Ark publications include several that are very relevant to the needs of visually handicapped children. *Choosing Toys and Activities for Handicapped Children* has sections on toys which stimulate touch and smell, and some suggestions to encourage babies and young children to use their residual vision. A toy library especially for visually handicapped

215

children is attached to the Research Centre for the Education of the Visually Handicapped, Birmingham.

The Good Toy Guide lists nine hundred toys that have been approved for their play value by the child care specialists of the Association. The toys are listed according to their particular value in encouraging a skill and there is an appendix detailing play equipment and toys specially designed for handicapped children as well as commercial toys which have been found to be particularly helpful.

Choosing toys

During recent years, increasing attention has been given to the part toys play in developing a child's skills and understanding. Children learn through play, and well-designed attractive toys appropriately chosen to encourage certain skills have special value for visually handicapped children who may receive little stimulus through their eyes. Severely visually handicapped children may indeed be very tentative in accepting any new toy, and will need to be shown how to play with it, perhaps several times, before they are ready to begin to enjoy playing with it by themselves. Even then, they may play with it quite differently to sighted children. A toy car, held upside down, with wheels that can be spun to make an intriguing noise is likely to be much more fun than the same car which, if pushed along the floor, disappears utterly.

Rough and ready rules when selecting toys are to choose ones that are shiny, or brightly coloured in hues the child is known to distinguish, which can be manipulated by the child and which will then give an immediate reward, and thus a sense of achievement. If he or she has little or no sight, the shape and texture of the toy are obviously important. Surprisingly, soft furry toys are often disliked by young blind children, though they may be more acceptable if they have a music box mechanism inside them. Models should be used with caution; it is far better to learn from life. As the author of *Children with a Severe Visual Defect* (RNIB) puts it: 'A duck to your baby is the sour smell of the pond, the gurgling sound of water and the familiar quack, nothing at all like a small plastic model.'

Help with choosing toys can be found in the booklet just quoted, and also in the pamphlet *Toys with a Purpose* by Heather Jones. This can be obtained through the RNIB Education Department and gives a great deal of help in choosing toys for children up to five years who have no useful sight. Mrs Head, an educational psychologist, is also happy to answer parents' queries on toys and to provide a reading list, a toy list (which is slanted towards the needs of each stage of a child's development, rather than towards a specific handicap) and a list of manufacturers. Requests should be sent to *Mrs Head, Education Psychology Service, 16 St Mary's Gate, Derby DE1 3JR.*

Play Helps (Roma Lear, Heinemann Health Books, 1977, £4.25) is a treasure house of ideas for cheap, easy, home-made toys that stimulate the five senses. The section on 'Making the Most of Touch' is the most relevant for blind children, with its ideas for ways of helping babies and toddlers to feel, making a 'feely corner', a feely caterpillar, and feely bingo and its description of a home-made 'open Sesame' board to enable children to become familiar with different door catches. Nevertheless, the sections devoted to the other four senses also contain much that is relevant to visually handicapped children, including ways of making a clanky pull-along, a noisy busy board, as well as how to play torch tag, the yummy yum game, and ways to go on a 'listening loiter'.

Commercially Available Toys

Many toys on sale in toy shops are suitable for visually handicapped children, and a careful reading of the catalogues issued by manufacturers should give parents plenty of ideas. Galt, Fisher-Price and Hestair Hope are excellent ones to study, preferably in conjunction with *The Good Toy Guide*. Toys which have proved their popularity with visually handicapped children include the Activity Centre (Fisher-Price), the Pop-Up-Cone Tree (Pedigree), Pop-up Toy (Galt), the Disco Dancing Mat (A.A. Hales) and Simon (Milton Bradley Ltd.). (The dancing mat is a large plastic mat with pressure pads; dance on the pads to create a tune. Simon is an electronic game where players have to follow a light and sound sequence which increases in difficulty.) Lists of commercial toys suitable for babies and pre-school children can be obtained from the RNIB Education Department.

Specially Designed Toys

The RNIB stocks a number of board games, including ludo, and a series of easy, raised outline jigsaw puzzles. An electronic ball (catalogue no. 9201), which emits a continuous high-pitched bleep so that it can easily be found, is also available from them. Full details can be found in their free *Games and Apparatus* catalogue. Some commercial manufacturers also stock toys designed for handicapped children, including the visually handicapped.

The ESA catalogue *Play Specials* is especially helpful and includes an excellent Cradle Play, several types of tactile boards and a non-tip safety baby walker, especially suitable for visually handicapped children. Contact *ESA, Fairview Road, Stevenage, Hertfordshire (tel. Stevenage (0438) 726383)*.

The *Four to Eight* catalogue includes finger tip dominoes, in which seven different materials are used so the dominoes can be matched by touch, and a large, easily handled version of noughts and crosses designed for children without sight. The address is *Medway House, Faircharm Industrial Estate, Evelyn Drive, Leicester, LE3 2BU (tel. Leicester (0533) 823353)*.

Toys to Encourage Residual Vision
Much depends on the vision of the individual child and his or her interests, but toys and games which have appealed to many partially sighted children include the wobbleglobe (Kiddicraft), and executive desk toys with moving silver balls. All brightly coloured toys are popular, and Escor Toys Ltd have an especially good catalogue of strongly made, wooden toys in gay colours. Their address is *Groveley Road, Christchurch, Dorset BH23 3RQ (tel. Christchurch (0202) 485834)*.

Older children have enjoyed Connect (Galt), a card game demanding the accurate matching of bold coloured lines, Swingball (Dunlop), an ideal outdoor bat and ball game in which the ball cannot be lost, and the many varieties of television games, especially table tennis. A list of toys and books and games suitable for partially sighted children from two years can be obtained through the RNIB Education Department and a booklet *Suggested Toys and Equipment* (20p) can be obtained from Mr Marshall (see page 215).

Toys for multiply handicapped children
Advice on toys for deaf/blind children is given by the National Association for Deaf/Blind and Rubella Handicapped who have a toy library of adapted toys at their Ealing centre (see page 255).

Huntercraft designs and markets 'special toys for special children'. The whole range has been designed and tested in hospitals and special schools, and each piece of equipment comes with full instructions on how it should be used. Items which have been found useful for the visually handicapped include the Huntercraft Feely Box to encourage discrimination between textures, and toys designed to capture visual attention such as the Defraction Box, which is a rotating cube with surfaces of brilliant patterned metallic paper which flash as it rotates, and the Zig Zag, which is designed to encourage the child to use his eyes from side to side as he follows the movement of a contrasting or sparkling disc along a wooden zig zag. Contact *Huntercraft, Sherbourne, Dorset (tel. Sherbourne (093581) 2288)*.

The RNIB booklet *Guidelines for Teachers and Parents of Visually Handicapped Children with Additional Handicaps* has many ideas for ingenious home-made toys, as well as listing commercial toys, which help a child develop and enjoy himself at the same time.

It would, however, be misleading to end a chapter on parents and children simply with a description of toys. People are more important than toys, and for the visually handicapped child above all there is no substitute for the company of the family. No toy can take the place of mother's conversation, her commentary as she does the household chores and her sharing of the tasks. The World Council for the Welfare of the Blind felt that this was so important that, for the International Year of the Child, they issued this parents' declaration:

We will play and spend as much time with you as we can. We will introduce you to as many games and activities as possible to help you use your hearing, your sense of touch and mobility so that your language, thought and imagination are enriched.

We will put lots of different objects and toys into your two hands, naming and describing them and telling you what they are for and how to play with them.

We will give you the opportunity to play with balls, dolls, vehicles, model kits, sand, paper, cardboard and plasticine, and do lots of collecting and sorting. We will let you use scissors, needles, thread, glue, hammers, nails and screws. Your toys will be painted in strongly contrasting colours and will not give you a wrong idea of the real thing.

We will make a safe play corner for you, and give you room to move about without hurting yourself. We will keep chairs and other furniture in fixed positions. If you do happen to collide with them occasionally, or make yourself dirty, we will not fuss too much or keep interfering with your play.

You will help us around the house. We shall have 'role' games, for example we will play 'shops' after we have gone shopping together at the real shops. Together, we will find sighted playmates and we will organise games with them and also take you to the local playground.

We shall be patient, even if you are clumsy. We will try and discover your interests and capacities and will help you and keep on helping you, to become as skilled and self-reliant as other children.

★ *My tea-trolley is like another hand to me. I use it to carry all sorts of things – not just dishes. I put my Perkins machine, typewriter and braille paper on it or even the talking book machine so that I can move them easily from one room to another. I don't push the trolley in front of me, I pull it with one hand so that the other hand is free to guide me. I even put the clothes basket on it and wheel it out into the garden when I want to put the laundry out to dry.*
(Miriam O'Donnell, Hastings)

★ *To amuse a blind toddler make maracas by putting split peas into an empty washing-up liquid container.*

★ *Encourage a blind toddler to wear shoes as soon as possible so that the child can start enjoying sound echoes as he walks about.*

★ *When going out for a walk with a blind child play stamping games as you pass the lamp posts on your way out – and try to get your child to find the lampposts again by stamping and listening carefully as he walks along the pavement on the way home.*
(Gill Hinds, Northampton)

Education

The education of visually handicapped children has been a matter of hot debate for some years. A Government Committee of Enquiry into the Education of Visually Handicapped Children reported in 1972 (the Vernon Report) and in 1978 *Special Education Needs: Report of the Committee of Enquiry into the Education of Handicapped Children and Young People* (the Warnock Report) was issued. At the time of writing, the Education Act 1981, based on the Warnock recommendations, has just received the Royal Assent, and is likely to be implemented during 1982/83. The new Act defines 'special educational needs' as covering learning difficulties which range from the minor and transient to the severe and complex. LEA's will be required to identify all children aged 2 years and over who have special educational needs and to arrange for their needs to be assessed. Based on the assessment, the LEA must then make a formal statement setting out the child's needs and the provision it proposes to make to meet them. LEA's will also have a duty to follow a similar procedure with children under 2 years of age if the parents so wish.

A formal assessment to record a child's 'special educational needs' does not mean that education in a special school will be automatically recommended. Indeed, the Act clearly states that such children should be educated in ordinary schools, so long as that is compatible with their receiving the education they need, the efficient education of the other children with whom they will be educated and the efficient use of resources.

The assessment and formal statement are obviously crucial factors in a handicapped child's career, and the Act lays a responsibility on LEA's to ensure that parents are consulted throughout the procedure. Parents will be able to see the statement in draft and, if they disagree with any aspect of it, they will have access to the experts who have provided the medical, educational and psychological evidence on which it is based. If parents are dissatisfied with the proposed provision, they have a right of appeal to the LEA's Appeals Committee, though that Committee's decision will not be binding on the LEA. There is a final right of appeal to the Secretary of State who is able to cancel or amend the statement after consulting the LEA. When a formal statement is made, parents will be given the name of a personal

221

contact to whom they can turn in the future if they need information and advice about their child's special educational needs.

Help and advice for parents, especially in regard to their child's placement and their rights of appeal, is offered by the Advisory Centre for Education. Their guide to the new Act entitled *The Law on Special Education* is available from 18 Victoria Park Square, London E2 9PB (01-980 4596) price £1.50 including postage.

Pre-School Help. At present, LEAs have the power (though not a duty) to provide pre-school education for visually handicapped children from the age of two years. The extent of this provision varies from authority to authority; it may include meeting the fees for under-fives attending a Sunshine Home.

Under the new Act, the Health Authority will be required to tell parents of any child under 5 years if, in their opinion, the child may have special educational needs, and also to inform the LEA. The Health Authority will also have a duty to let parents know of any voluntary organisation which may be able to help them meet those needs. Parents of visually handicapped children should therefore be informed of the RNIB Education Advisory Service (page 214). If, following assessment, pre-school education is recommended, the LEA will then have a duty to provide this.

Local provision for visually handicapped children varies greatly, and the LEA, RNIB adviser, health visitor or local social services department should be able to give information. Very occasionally there will be a special playgroup or nursery class. Sometimes ordinary playgroups are able to accept a visually handicapped child. Social services departments register all playgroups in their area and, therefore, are well able to advise parents which local playgroups are most likely to meet their child's needs. An alternative source of help is the Pre-School Playgroups Association, which encourages its groups to cater for children with 'special needs', and has a national advisor who is able to give help and advice on any aspect of handicapped children and playgroups. Linked to the Pre-School Playgroups Association are 'opportunity groups'. These, unlike playgroups which usually cater for children aged between three and five years, accept handicapped children from birth, have a high proportion of handicapped children and a much higher ratio of helpers to children – one-to-one is the general aim.

Special or ordinary school?

The phrase in the new Act 'efficient use of resources' suggests that integration is neither an easy nor a cheap alternative to segregated education. To be effective, especially perhaps for very severely visually handicapped children, a heavy input of expensive and scarce resources is needed. The bleak warning of the government in 1981 is that if additional manpower and funds are required these 'will become available only as the economic situation permits'.

However, it is unlikely that the new legislation will end the current arguments as to whether it is best for visually handicapped children to attend a local school, being given special help where necessary, or attend a special school, geared exclusively to their needs, but which is likely to be so far away from home that they will, at best, be weekly boarders. It seems likely that this either/or question is far too simple; both systems have their advantages and disadvantages. The needs of individual visually handicapped children vary so much that there cannot be one simple answer. In addition, some children may need to move between one type of education and the other at different stages of their development.

Attendance at an ordinary school is dependent on the willingness of the head teacher to accept a visually handicapped pupil, and in turn that willingness will generally be dependent on the local resources available to provide the essential 'back-up' facilities. Other key factors include the ability of the visually handicapped child, the degree of residual vision and the use he or she can make of low vision aids, including closed-circuit television, and the amount of support received at home. Examples of successful integration can be found in *Towards Integration: a study of blind and partially sighted children in ordinary schools* (Jameson, Parlett and Pocklington, National Federation for Education Research) which is also available in braille. It is noticeable, however, that all the children in this survey had some useful vision.

Staff resources

About half of the local education authorities in the country employ a specialist teacher/adviser who is professionally trained and experienced in the needs of visually handicapped children. In addition, some special schools act as a resource centre for their area. A notable example is Lickey Grange School, Birmingham, which, as the resource centre for the Midland Region, offers an information service, short or long-term assessment of children's educational needs, holiday courses for teachers, advice on aids and equipment and a modest braille and large print service. The Deputy Head, Mr R. Mayho, has oversight of resource provision and can give further details.

Unfortunately, it is not unknown for teachers in ordinary schools to find a pupil with poor sight and to discover that there is little advice to help them in their own area. One source of help is the RNIB Education Advisory Service (see page 214) but there is also a growing selection of publications to meet this need.

Notes for Teachers of Visually Handicapped Children not in Special Classes (Disabled Living Foundation) is a straightforward guide to sources of help, useful books and equipment.

Guidelines for Teachers in Ordinary Schools (RNIB) gives imaginative advice and suggests solutions to everyday problems. Publications obtainable through the Association for the Education and Welfare of the Visually-handicapped include *The Vocabulary of the Young Blind School Child* M. Tobin, *24 Selected Articles* (Teaching methods for different subjects) and the Teachers Handbook and print text of the *Family Books Reading Scheme* (braille learning for 5–9 year olds), and a revised edition of the handbook, *Children with Partial Sight*. Large print log tables are published when demand warrants it.

Visually Handicapped Children and Young People (E.K. Chapman, Routledge & Kegan Paul) has a section on visually handicapped children in ordinary schools, but the whole book is a mine of information for the non-specialist teacher.

The Partially Sighted Society is also building up a stock of information regarding partially sighted children.

Special schools
Increasingly, schools for the visually handicapped are encouraging their pupils to join in the activities of sighted schools. Children from St Vincent's School for the Blind and Partially Sighted in Liverpool attend a local sighted school for some 'O' and 'A' level subjects, and at Tapton Mount School, Sheffield, which takes blind children from five to twelve years, selected pupils attend a local comprehensive school for secondary education, whilst living in a hostel on the campus of Tapton Mount.

All special schools for blind and partially sighted children are run by local authorities or by voluntary societies. Details of blind and partially sighted schools are listed in the free RNIB booklet *Education of Blind Children*. Further details of schools for partially sighted children can be obtained from the Partially Sighted Society.

Admission to a special school
As has already been discussed (page 221) it is likely that procedures for admission to special school are likely to change in 1982/3. At present, local education authorities follow a procedure whereby forms are completed by the child's head teacher if he or she is already at school, and the school doctor (or, for a child not at school, the Area Health Authority Specialist in Community Medicine, Child Health), and then an educational psychologist sees both reports, before also completing one.

Parents should be consulted all through this process, so that when a final decision is made by the LEA they can feel that they have been partners in the decision-making process, bringing their own intimate knowledge of their child to supplement the expertise of the professionals.

Nursery schools
For blind children whose needs cannot be adequately met in their own homes, there are four Sunshine Home nursery schools, run by the RNIB, where children may be admitted – after consultation with one of the RNIB consultant paediatricians – for long or short periods according to their individual needs. It is rare for a child to be admitted to a Sunshine Home before the age of three; and they usually stay until the age of six or seven, or a little older if their development is slower due to additional handicaps. Sunshine Homes may also accept young blind children for an assessment period, or simply to enable the rest of the family to enjoy a short holiday. Information about Sunshine Homes can be obtained from the RNIB's Education Department.

Primary schools
Primary schools for blind children are residential, though day pupils are accepted and weekly boarding is common. Partially sighted children are often placed in special units in their own locality, though there are some residential schools for partially sighted children.

Secondary schools

Secondary schools for blind children are often combined with primary schools and thus cater for children from five to sixteen years. Secondary education is still selective for blind children and there are two grammar schools: Worcester College for boys and Chorleywood College for girls. Schools for partially sighted children are more numerous, so partially sighted children are more likely to attend daily, though inevitably some children have to be boarders because of the travelling involved.

Sixteen-plus

Vocational assessment

There are two assessment centres, Hethersett, Reigate (RNIB) and the Queen Alexandra College, Birmingham (BRIB) which cater for blind school leavers and partially sighted students whose sight is likely to deteriorate. The aim of these centres is to act as a bridge between the world of school and the world of work. Both centres assess the aptitudes and interests of students and guide them towards suitable training and employment, but also concentrate on the acquisition of daily living skills. In addition, the Queen Alexandra College offers a number of pre-vocational courses which can be developed into vocational courses, tailored to the needs of individual students and lasting between six and twelve months. From both centres, students can go out direct to employment or into 'training on the job', though some will join the courses described in Chapter 4. There are no equivalent centres specifically for partially sighted school leavers, though some receive further training at Skill Centres, admission being arranged by their Disablement Resettlement Officer found at the Job Centre. The establishment of a specialist centre for these young people is one of the concerns of the Partially Sighted Society, which is also engaged in research aiming to identify occupations particularly suited to the partially sighted.

Further education

The Royal National College for the Blind, Hereford, offers commercial training to blind and partially sighted students over the age of 16. The normal course lasts for three years and aims to achieve the RSA Elementary Typewriting Certificate in four or five terms and

Advanced Typewriting or Advanced Audio-Typewriting by the end of the course. Instruction is also given in braille shorthand and speeds of 120 wpm are aimed at. All students study a core curriculum which includes braille (if required), English, arithmetic, mobility and living skills, as well as the opportunity to take 'O' levels, and, for students with the necessary aptitude, 'A' levels. Students are given experience in telephony and opportunities of work experience away from the College. The aim is that they should be able to live independently and to obtain posts in open employment on leaving College. There is no upper age limit. Applicants are normally assessed at the College before being accepted.

The Royal National College offers General Studies courses leading to qualifications for entry into universities and colleges, including the North London School of Physiotherapy. There are also courses for full-time musicians, including 'A' level, the LRAM and the LGSM Piano Teachers' Diploma. New computer studies courses are being introduced in 1981; these will include GCE courses and the City and Guilds Basic Certificate in Computer Programming.

The Queen Alexandra College, Birmingham, also offers a range of further education courses as well as the vocational courses detailed on pages 46–47. Subjects include household maintenance, daily living skills, and adult literacy – a course in all means of communication devised specifically for the visually handicapped.

Higher education

An increasing number of blind and partially sighted students are now pursuing full-time courses of further and higher education. In 1980 there were 209 such students studying in ninety-one different institutions, as well as ninety-eight students enrolled in the Open University. These students are the special concern of the RNIB Education Department, which issues notes on the library and allied sources available for students and notes for the guidance of academic staff concerned with visually handicapped students. The Association of Blind and Partially Sighted Teachers and Students acts as a pressure group for such students and offers consultation and advice. The National Bureau for Handicapped Students also aims to improve opportunities in further and higher education for all handicapped students and provides information and advice on facilities and services available, holds conferences and publishes a quarterly newsletter, *Educare*.

Financial help

A student with a visual handicap inevitably has to incur extra expenses. LEAs can now increase the standard student grant, if a student can show that he has to incur additional expense because of his handicap. This extra allowance was fixed at up to £235 per annum in 1981.

In addition, the RNIB is prepared to make grants, initially of up to £400, to cover costs of material or services such as braille equipment, typewriters, tape recorders, payment of readers. This grant can be extended by a further £300 according to the student's needs. The grant is made in the form of a credit account against which these items may be charged.

The Hampshire and Isle of Wight Educational Trust for the Blind awards blind or partially sighted students travel, book, pocket and readers' allowances and assists with the provision of special equipment and with general expenses. It does not limit its help to students from Hampshire and the Isle of Wight, though students there have priority. Address: *48 Stubbington Avenue, Portsmouth, PO2 0HY (tel. Portsmouth (0705) 61717)*.

The North Wales Trust Fund offers financial assistance to blind and partially sighted young people under twenty-one years of age who need help in their education – perhaps by the provision of items such as braille writers or typewriters, which cannot be provided by statutory funds. Address: *325 High Street, Bangor, Gwynedd LL57 1YB (tel. Bangor (0248) 53604)*.

Continuing education

The Open University

A number of blind and partially sighted people have graduated through the Open University. The Open University is especially sensitive to the needs of disabled students generally, and offers a counselling service to help them deal with the practical problems they may encounter throughout their study period. Prospective students who wish to find out more about the university can borrow recordings of the current *Guide for Applicants for BA Degree Courses* and the *BA Degree Handbook* from the RNIB Student Tape Library.

Special facilities for visually handicapped students include the opportunity to attend a weekend preparatory study course which is arranged by the Open University. Here new students have the chance to meet counselling staff and tutors and share the experience of other blind people who have completed degree courses either with the Open University or at other universities. A number of Open University course materials and set books are issued on tape; full details can be obtained from the RNIB or the Open University. Anyone interested should contact *Richard Tomlinson, Adviser on the Education of the Disabled, The Open University, Walton Hall, Milton Keynes, Buckinghamshire MK7 6AA (tel. Milton Keynes (0908) 74066)*.

Correspondence courses

The Hadley School for the Blind, Illinois, USA, offers a wide variety of courses on cassette, and in braille. Subjects vary from a rapid braille reading course to first aid without fear, creative writing, classical Greek and typing, a total of 135 courses. All the courses are free to the students but, because of the great expense involved for the school, students have a responsibility not to enrol lightly. Full details of all courses and an enrolment form are available in the Students Information Bulletin, in large print, or in any of the media mentioned above, on request from *The Hadley School for the Blind, 700 Elm Street, Winnetka, Illinois 60093, USA*.

Adult education

Many visually handicapped people join in the evening and day classes arranged by adult education departments, and the Workers Educational Association. The local library will be able to give details of classes held locally. Sometimes special classes for the visually handicapped are held, when it is felt that more personal tuition is required than could be given in a large class of sighted students. Visually handicapped adults who are interested in joining any group but are hesitant about their ability to keep up with the class, should discuss the matter with the adult education officer responsible – the name and address will be known at the local library.

Most tutors welcome the challenge of a visually handicapped student, though they will need guidance from him or her as to exactly what extra help is needed. Once the needs are identified, it is a rare class or tutor that does not provide a volunteer only too willing to offer help by tape recording, or making diagrams, or by reading aloud.

(For a discussion of the educational opportunities for multiply

229

handicapped blind children and young people, see Chapter 19, *Additional disabilities,* pages 255–56.)

Further Reading
Higher Education Preview.
Facilities and Course Options for Visually Handicapped Students in UK Universities and Polytechnics. The Partially Sighted Society 1981 £1.

★ *A partially-sighted child should always have a torch (or a torch magnifier) and a thick black marking pen in his pocket or school bag. The first are for his own use when he finds himself trying to see something in a poorly-lit area; and the second is to lend his teacher when his work is being marked in class.*

★ *Students will find revision easier if notes are brailled on different sizes of paper, according to their importance. Use small size braille paper for notes that have to be carried around a great deal.*
(Kevin Mulhern)

18 Help for the very elderly

The usual age at which people are registered as blind is between eighty and eighty-nine years. This fact is more disturbing when it is realised that the number of people over seventy-five in the population as a whole is steadily rising, and the number over the age of eighty-five is expected to increase from 464,000 in 1980 to 692,000 in 1995. The commonest cause of visual disability in this age group is macular degeneration, closely followed by cataract. Therefore, for a very high proportion of people on the blind register, 'blindness' consists of failing vision, rather than total loss of sight, during the closing years of life.

At an advanced age, visual disability is rarely the only handicap. An individual may be so preoccupied with the aches and pains of arthritis, or the breathlessness due to heart trouble, that failing sight may seem to be the least urgent of many problems. Recent studies have indicated that only 60 per cent of visually disabled adults living at home are likely to have had a specialist examination of their eyes, and of these over half will be more than seventy-five years of age. The blind and partially sighted registers are now acknowledged to be far from comprehensive. The implications of these stark facts are only just being recognised by many blind welfare agencies, which explains why so often the aids mentioned in this book call for an alert mind, nimble fingers and acute hearing with registration as a prerequisite for services.

Registration as a time of crisis

For the very elderly, continuing independence is often very precarious. Registration may cause the balance to be tipped disastrously, and both helpers and helped need to be convinced that this crisis can be overcome. The old are by their very natures resilient; they have lived through two world wars, economic depression and unemployment, and have experienced all the joys and sorrows that are intermingled in a long life. The strengths derived from these experiences can enable them to cope with this new setback, provided that courage is not sapped and self-confidence destroyed by the well-meaning attitudes of those around them.

Snatching away the mildewing loaf with the comment 'You can't eat that' may prevent an upset stomach, but the damage to morale is not repaired so easily. By working alongside – for example, sorting out the bread bin together whilst discussing the shortcomings of the modern bakery industry – one can help constructively. In the same way, appropriate help given quickly at the time of crisis – a signature guide, a large print dial for the telephone, a radio or even a white stick – has virtue far beyond the intrinsic value of the aid; it conveys the message, 'You're not alone, and we believe you can manage.'

Can sight be improved?
It is clear that, among the very elderly, the identification of those with poor sight cannot be left to the 'experts', for without help, they are unlikely ever to reach the professionals. Anyone can check whether an old lady has cancelled her newspaper order solely because she is weary of reading about gloom and doom, or because she just cannot see the print clearly.

If an elderly person gives up doing close work in the evenings or on dark days, this is generally an indication that the lighting needs improving (see Chapter 9). A visit to the optician for new spectacles can prove helpful at ninety years of age and over. Ophthalmic opticians can make home visits under the NHS when this is essential, though it may take persistence to find an optician willing to do this. If new spectacles will not help, the optician will notify the patient's family doctor, who can then arrange for an examination at hospital by an ophthalmologist. Nowadays it is not unknown for patients in their mid-nineties to have their cataracts removed and later be able to read their hundredth birthday telegram from the Queen!

Yet the fact must be faced that, for many elderly people, the last years will be spent in a world of blurred outlines and indistinct faces, where objects are never quite where they seem to be, where kerbs disappear and the depth of steps cannot be judged accurately. To be hesitant and slow-moving in such a situation, resistant to change and new ideas, and cautious in contact with strangers – all these are natural and self-protecting reactions which would-be helpers should appreciate when they are bubbling over with ideas which might very well solve the person's problems.

Living independently
Chapters 5 and 6 deal with methods by which some of the problems

involved in daily living can be tackled or shared. Many very elderly visually handicapped people continue to live alone; sometimes they even care for a handicapped spouse, regardless of all difficulties. Determination rather than disability seems to be the key factor.

Keeping warm
Elderly visually handicapped people who move slowly are inevitably liable to suffer from the cold. The twin fears of expensive fuel bills and of accidental fire also combine to make them particularly at risk. It is, therefore, important not to undermine self-confidence when discussing heating. Coal fires can look very dangerous to the outsider, but many visually handicapped people manage them perfectly safely; a lifetime's experience is not wiped out because eyesight has dimmed. The provision of a good fireguard, or information about smokeless fuels which will not suddenly send out a shower of sparks, are more positive ways of helping than immediately suggesting a different method of heating.

If, however, there is a real fear of fire, then help may be needed to provide heaters of the types mentioned on page 68. For example, old oil heaters, which are difficult to fill and easy to knock over, can be very dangerous indeed, but may be used for reasons of economy. Grants to meet the cost of buying a safer appliance may be available from any of the following sources in cases of financial hardship: the Department of Health and Social Security (see leaflet SB 17 – 'Help with Heating Costs'); the local branch of Age Concern; and, for registered blind or partially sighted people, the local voluntary society for the blind, or one of the larger national charities (see page 42). A small weekly grant towards increased running costs may also be made by one of these charities.

A room thermometer is sometimes useful in persuading elderly people to keep an appliance switched on; otherwise they may feel that by switching on they are weakly giving in to their 'feelings'. Large thermometers, with very clear print (black on white) are available from Habitat by mail order, and a tactile wall thermometer is stocked by the RNIB. A thermometer will also provided useful evidence when applying for a heating allowance (see page 37).

People who have to spend much of their time in an armchair often feel chilly when the room seems comfortably warm to others. For sheer comfort, the old-fashioned hot water bottle is hard to beat. An especially suitable model for visually handicapped people who have to fill their own is the Dunlop Cosimax; this has a very wide neck, making it easier to fill, and a stopper cover big enough to fold back over the knuckles to protect them from splashes. It is available throughout the United Kingdom from good class chemists. If necessary, it can be obtained by post from the Mail Order Department of *Harrods Ltd, PO Box 372, Knightsbridge, London SW1X 7XL.*

Many visually handicapped people cope with filling hot water bottles by using a funnel. A particularly suitable one is the 'Safety' funnel made by Arthur Douglas Ltd, which has a collar around the top of the stem to allow air to escape to reduce the danger of hot water bubbling over the top of the funnel however fast it is poured (see page 87 for address).

Electric heating pads (designed to be used by someone sitting in a chair) which can even be wrapped round an aching joint, avoid all the difficulties involved in filling hot water bottles. But they do offer another hazard – that of tripping over the flex, so the armchair should be carefully positioned in relation to the socket.

For warmth at night, over- and under- electric blankets are well known and are easy to control, being designed for manipulation in |the dark! If underneath warmth is needed all through the night, the only suitable type is a low-voltage underblanket.

People who dislike the idea of electric heating in their bed may find a fleecy underblanket is the answer to their problem. These not only provide all-night warmth, but are helpful in preventing pressure sores when the user is bedridden. The most luxurious are natural sheepskin, but these need very careful laundering; others have a synthetic backing to the fleece which makes washing easier, and another type has synthetic fleece and synthetic backing and so is very easy to wash. Small squares can be purchased for use on a chair. Details of blankets and heating pads can be obtained from the Disabled Living Foundation.

Living with relatives
It is always sad when people have to give up their own home and move in with relatives, however welcoming and caring these may be. On both sides there is likely to be a good deal of apprehension, and it is often helpful for both parties to discuss the issues involved – and the alternatives open – with a social worker before a decision is made. If the old person is being discharged from hospital, the hospital social worker is a good person to consult.

Once the decision is made, the first section of Chapter 10 becomes very relevant. The stress of moving and the new surroundings are likely to be very confusing, and visually handicapped people may feel their sight is, if anything, worse, especially if they have no mental picture of their new home. The route from bedroom to toilet may be crucial, and a rail along the passage wall to act as a guide might relieve some anxiety. If space can be found, the room should be large enough and warm enough for use as a bed-sitting room – a place to retreat to in order to listen to radio or talking book, and where privacy is ensured with the certainty that no one is watching. This room should be very much the visually handicapped person's kingdom, to be arranged as he or she desires it, even though the arrangement may not be aesthetically agreeable to others. Some blind people love a multitude of ornaments and photographs, while others prefer a regimented order which may give the room a bleak and spartan air. Where the elderly guest shares the living room, a low vision aid (page 111) may enable television to be watched without others' view of the screen being blocked; for the hard of hearing, the listening devices mentioned on page 246 may be especially welcome.

As important as providing a comfortable environment, however, is the need to help the newcomer feel at home. It is no kindness at all to insist on doing everything, for no one wants to be a passenger. Modern kitchen gadgets may be unfamiliar, but vegetables can be prepared in the old-fashioned way and it is still a help for the busy housewife if she has only to check the potatoes are all peeled, rather than do the whole job herself. Some elderly visually handicapped people become shoe-polishers-in-chief, others are teachers-extraordinary, for what child can resist reading aloud to someone who really wants to know what the letter says? Cleaning the cutlery, polishing the brass, dealing with the plain ironing, even becoming senior dishcloth knitter to the family and neighbourhood gives status and self-respect. When a listener to *In Touch* enquired how one occupied one's mind when 90 years of age and housebound, suggestions from blind people ranged from crocheting in bright wool on a contrasting background, to recording reminiscences of early life on tape for the benefit of younger members of the family, or oral history groups.

Giving relatives a break
With the best will in the world, both carers and cared-for need a

respite from each other occasionally! The local blind club should be able to meet some of the social needs of the very elderly and frail, and if it has a warm and welcoming atmosphere it can give the visually handicapped person a great deal of pleasure, companionship and interest. Relatives who are at work all day may find their local social services department can arrange day care at a nearby old people's home or day centre, and a stay in the same home may be arranged to enable the other members of the family to take their annual holiday. Many blind homes run by voluntary organisations (see page 199) also have holiday beds for short-term guests, and a local social worker should be able to advise appropriately. When nursing care is needed the doctor or health visitor may be able to arrange a short-stay bed in a local geriatric hospital. When nursing is becoming a very heavy burden a 'six weeks in, six weeks out' scheme is sometimes available.

Home nursing
Statutory services are briefly discussed on pages 57–8. There are many ways, however, to make life pleasanter for a blind invalid without professional help. Meals in bed can be difficult to manage unless there is a stable surface to take the dishes. This can be provided by a bed-table, but even an ordinary tray can be used more easily if the plates are held in position by non-slip mats.

Food guards, which are simple plastic collars which clip around ordinary household plates, prevent food being pushed off the edge. Manoy plates, attractively designed in Melaware, are cleverly shaped with a sloping base and deep rim at one end which actually helps a person to get the food on the spoon. Suction egg-cups will stop the breakfast egg sliding around. A plastic meal tray, which can be clamped by its suction feet to tray or table, is available; it comes complete with a deep and a shallow dish, and a beaker, all of which fit snugly into its moulded recesses.

On the bedside cupboard, a glass of water is more likely to be visible if the glass is in a brightly coloured plastic holder (Pyrex drink-up) or in a stable, brightly coloured Melaware mug (Rosti). Hot drinks throughout the day can be poured very easily by the invalid himself if a vacuum flask with a pump dispenser is put on a non-slip mat by the bed.

Attractive nightdresses always make the patient feel better; and if they are easy to put on and present no problems when using the toilet, they are doubly attractive. Styles with a button-through front and a

236

wrap-over back meet both these requirements and can be purchased in pretty nylon or polyester materials.

An audible clock (page 73) may be easier to use than a tactile model and is small enough to go in a pyjama pocket. The many things that can so easily be lost in bed, or be out of reach, can be stowed safely in a shoe-tidy. This useful set of pockets, generally found in haberdashery departments, can be hooked on the near-side of the bedside cupboard or the top section can be anchored firmly between mattress and base.

Toilet needs may cause problems. Commodes can generally be borrowed via the community nurse, social worker or local Red Cross branch. Apart from standard bedpans, there are specially designed urinals for women and the Suba-Seal would be especially helpful for a blind person as it is non-spill. It consists of a small shallow plastic dish with a capped hollow handle through which it is emptied. A non-spill adaptor, made of rigid nylon with a rubber sleeve will fit most male urinals and is sold in packets of five by *Chas. F. Thackray, Ltd, Viaduct Road, Leeds LS4 2BR (tel. Leeds (0532) 31862)*.

Advice on all the special aids listed in this section should be available through local social services departments and many may be available on loan or on trial. The Disabled Living Foundation can also give further details, including prices and names of suppliers.

Confined to bed?
Filling in the time is often a problem, especially when long periods are spent in bed or in bed-side chair. Listening to the radio is always a standby, and the push-button set described on page 161 solves many difficulties of programme location. The tape recording services mentioned in Chapter 13 are likely to be enjoyed. A number of the games stocked by the RNIB can be played in bed, as counters have been replaced by pegs (see page 86). The tantalisingly difficult Bramah puzzle (RNIB catalogue no. 9185) has given hours of enjoyable mental challenge, especially to those who are anxious to reassure themselves that their brain is still active. Braillists have fewer problems, of course, but some very elderly people have pleasure in discovering Moon (page 146) and discovering that, although they may not succeed in reading fluently, they gain satisfaction in learning enough to identify giant Moon playing cards or to make out already familiar pieces of Scripture. Hand writing is possible and the Portland Frame (RNIB catalogue no. 9166) in particular provides a very firm surface for writing.

A good light over the top of the bed, or clipped on the headboard, may make other activities possible. Some simple crafts may be enjoyed and those who want to knit for a good cause will find that the Save the Children Fund is always glad to receive knitted squares – details of measurements can be obtained from the Fund direct or from any local organiser.

A bed placed alongside, or at an angle to, the window rather than facing it, will enable the patient to see better – especially if he or she suffers from cataract and is dazzled by direct sunlight.

A sturdy reading stand, such as that made by Joncare, will take a large print book, and its suction feet clamp firmly to bed table or tray. Contact *Joncare Ltd, Radley Road, Abingdon, Oxfordshire (tel. Abingdon (0236) 28120)*.

Going to hospital
It is not safe to assume that all hospital staff will automatically appreciate the problems of a visually handicapped patient. Relatives or friends should certainly make it clear on admission the kind of visual problems the patient has, and the help usually needed. Otherwise, there is the possibility of a patient's being regarded as a 'fractured femur', for example, and – especially if there is some guiding sight – the visual disability may be completely overlooked. Then the danger is that he or she may also be regarded as 'a bit dim' or 'confused' because either the wrong response or no response at all is made to the comments of the passing nurse. It is not unknown for a cup of tea left on a bed table to be removed later without the patient ever realising it was there, simply because the tea-lady did not know the patient could not see.

If sight is very poor indeed, it would be helpful to suggest to the staff that they should indicate their presence, and say what they intend to do before they actually do it. It is reassuring to be told, for example, that the curtains have been pulled round the bed before the examination starts. Unless it is very carefully and slowly explained, moving a blind person with a hoist can be most terrifying for anyone who has not been able to watch other patients being lifted comfortably by it. Nor does a voice from the end of the bed, however kindly the words, give the reassurance of a touch of the hand, or the comfort of an arm round the shoulders. It is also easy to forget that irritation, hurry and impatience are also easily sensed through touch, and when the patient cannot see how busy and anxious the nurse is, any feelings of vulnerability are reinforced.

Some blind people feel that some of these problems could be overcome if beds were marked to indicate that the patient could not see – one blind man solved this problem by persuading a nurse to write 'blind' in large letters by his name on the bedhead. Not all blind people would wish to advertise their handicap in this way, but even so might well appreciate an opportunity of avoiding the embarrassments almost bound to occur in situations when many different staff are attending to them.

A life-saver for me has been a small pocket made from material which I fasten, by safety-pins, to the mattress on my bed near my pillow. I use it to keep my pills, eye drops, handkerchief etc. which I need to use during the night.
(D.E. Anderson, Bexhill-on-Sea)

Wear an apron with two large pockets under your coat when you go out shopping. Keep your money in three separate purses which can be easily distinguished by touch. e.g. a smooth purse for notes, a crinkly one for silver and a soft, silky purse for copper. This way your hands are free to cope with shopping and money is safe.
(May Rainer, Bracknell)

Put a brightly coloured tablecloth on the table. It is much easier to see white cups and saucers against a plain deep orange or blue tablecloth.
(Doris Probert, Carshalton)

19 Additional disabilities

Diabetes
Diabetes is a complex condition and a minority of diabetics find that their eyesight is affected. However, when one looks at the blind population as a whole, diabetes is a major cause of blindness amongst those of working age, and many in this group are insulin dependent. Visually handicapped people who develop diabetes late in life are more likely to find that the condition can be controlled by dietary means alone or by diet and tablets. A number of aids have been developed to enable visually handicapped people to cope with their own injections, but it is sad for both groups that so little information is available to them. For example, information on dietary control in large print or on tape is virtually non-existent so that the elderly visually handicapped have little opportunity to remind themselves of the information given verbally at the diabetic clinic.

Insulin therapy
Most visually handicapped diabetics have become accustomed to administer their own injections, but when their sight deteriorates they will need to acquire some further skill. As always, order and method are vital. When preparing for an injection, all items needed should be placed in order where they may be found easily. Insulin bottles should be lightly shaken before every injection to check that there is sufficient for the injection. If two different kinds of insulin are used, one bottle should have an embossed symbol, adhesive tape or an elastic band. The Hypoguard complete insulin user's case encourages a tidy mind! This is a rigid plastic container with a snap-on lid, designed to hold all the items for an injection. It is compact enough to fit into a large pocket or handbag, and is particularly suitable for use when travelling.

Measuring insulin doses: Distinguishing the calibrations on the syringe is the first problem. Some disposable syringes have very clear markings, but these may vary between different batches. Good lighting should improve visibility; the best results are often achieved when the lighting source is behind the syringe barrel, but the beam must be carefully directed so that it does not also shine into the eyes. A clip-on magnifier can be purchased from Hypoguard, but it is likely to help

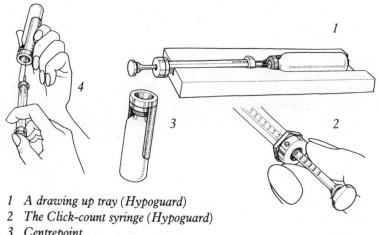

1 A drawing up tray (Hypoguard)
2 The Click-count syringe (Hypoguard)
3 Centrepoint
4 Drawing up with Centrepoint

only those who do not require a high magnification. Lenses giving up to eight times magnification and which leave the hands free to deal with the syringe include the lobster pot model (illustrated on page 109) and jeweller's loupes which are gripped in the eye in the same way as a monocle. When magnification cannot help, a pre-set syringe (available on prescription) can solve the problem, provided that a sighted person checks the setting at least once a week to make sure that it has not slipped slightly. For complete independence, visually handicapped diabetics often prefer a Hypoguard click-count syringe which, unlike the pre-set syringe, has the advantage that it can be used for mixed doses of insulin.

The calibrations on a click-count syringe are marked by grooves on the spindle, and there is a distinctive resistance and click at each point. Either smooth or clicking action can be selected, and there is a tactile indicator for this. The smooth action should be selected when injecting air into the bottle, when expelling air from the syringe, and before the actual injection. The dose can also be checked by feeling the number of exposed grooves with a finger nail. It is, of course, essential that the user has a sensitive touch, as well as natural dexterity and a methodical mind, if this syringe is to be handled safely and confidently. It is strongly recommended that the click-count syringe should be used under medical or nursing supervision until the technique has been completely mastered. This syringe can be purchased in

1 ml. or 2 ml. sizes, but it is not available on prescription, though some hospital diabetic clinics may supply it out of their discretionary funds.

Drawing up the insulin dose: The main problem lies in inserting the syringe needle through the tiny rubber seal at the centre of the cap of the insulin bottle, as clumsiness leads to bent or blunted needles. 'Centrepoint' (illustration on page 241) is a stainless steel needle guide in the shape of a funnel which clips over the cap of the insulin bottle to guide the needle to the centre of the seal. This gadget has the advantage that it allows the needle to be inserted into the bottle in the conventional manner. It is designed by a blind man and comes in two sizes to fit both short, squat (Boots, Burroughs Wellcome, Allen and Hanbury) and the tall, thin (Nova) 10 ml. bottles in which insulin is usually dispensed. Centrepoint can be purchased from the inventor *R.N. Beard, 40 Richmond Close, Calmore, Southampton SO4 2TH (tel. Totton (0703) 868703.*

The Hypoguard plastic location tray also illustrated on page 241 serves the same purpose. It is essentially a mould into which can be slotted a 1 ml. or 2 ml. syringe (including the click-count and the pre-set syringes) and any normal insulin bottle. Bottle and syringe are then held in correct alignment to ensure the needle pierces the sealing disc. This method enables the piercing to be done comfortably on the level, but then of course syringe and bottle have to be carefully removed from the mould and the bottle inverted for the drawing up of the insulin to be completed.

The injection: Though the technique learned at the clinic should be practised as far as possible, the following suggestions may help visually handicapped diabetics. Having prepared for an injection, it is sometimes difficult to insert the needle into the pinched-up mound of skin at the right place, at the correct angle, and to the correct depth. The little finger of the hand holding the syringe can be placed on the injection site to act as a guide and gauge the amount of penetration. It is most important for the visually handicapped diabetic to use the correct size of needle, i.e. 26 gauge by ½" or ⅝". Only if the needle is sharp, pushed in quickly, and inserted to the correct depth, will an effective and pain-free injection be achieved. An ingenious device, the Hypoguard Automatic Injector, makes it easy for diabetics, sighted or blind, to overcome most of the self-injection problems. It consists of an inner tube, which is fitted between the needle and syringe before drawing up the insulin, and an outer sliding sleeve, which is clipped into position, concealing the needle, immediately prior to the injection. This device enables the user to achieve a virtually painless injection, at the correct depth, using one hand only, in any of the seven alternative injection sites (including the normally inaccessible upper arms). An adaptor is included for use if the longer (⅝″) needle is used. There is no need to pinch up the skin, it can be used at almost any angle and the extra length of the instrument is quickly accepted by most people.

Self-monitoring
Independence in checking urine for glucose level is now possible. A battery-operated audio urine meter is available from Hypoguard and sometimes through diabetic clinics. Operation is simple: a diastix is placed in a socket and the instrument communicates the result of the test by means of a buzzer code, and will report one of six conditions: 0 per cent, $^1/_{10}$ per cent, ¼ per cent, ½ per cent, 1 per cent and 2 per cent. Audible versions of the increasingly widely used blood glucose monitors are not available, but some brands do have very clear large print digital read-outs. At the time of writing this is an area of rapid change and prospective purchasers should seek up-to-date advice from their diabetic clinic or the British Diabetic Association.

Diastixs can be obtained free on prescription, but unfortunately this is not true of either type of monitor. In view of the considerable expenditure alone, it would be wise to seek medical advice before purchase; but the fact that reliable readings are pointless unless correct use can be made of the information gained makes medical advice in the early stages essential.

Information service
The British Diabetic Association offers advice and help to all diabetics, and is particularly anxious that the visually handicapped should not be excluded. The Association's bi-monthly newspaper, *Balance*, is recorded on compact cassette for any visually handicapped diabetic joining the association (annual subscription 50p). No charge is made for the cassette: members listen to it and return it post-free to the BDA. *Balance* is full of interesting items: recipes, a correspondence column, details of diabetic problems and articles about diabetes.

Understanding Diabetes, a sixty-minute cassette, which includes inter-

243

views with a consultant physician and a dietician, and discusses both mild and insulin-dependent types of diabetes can be purchased from Hypoguard.

A free braille pamphlet, *Living with Diabetes – a Guide for Insulin-Dependent Diabetics*, is available from the RNIB as is a braille cookery book entitled *Measure for Measure*.

Holidays: Interesting new developments are the annual holidays organised by the British Diabetic Association. Designed for the older insulin-dependent adult, they aim to give participants a better understanding of diabetes, enable them to become independent regarding injections and to work out interesting and appetising menus within the limits of their diet. All this is done in a holiday atmosphere and setting, yet with easy access to medical and dietetic counselling. Full details can be obtained from the BDA.

Hearing difficulties
Anyone with a hearing problem should in the first instance consult his or her doctor. If a hearing aid is likely to help, the patient will be referred to an ear, nose and throat specialist who can prescribe a hearing aid free of charge through the National Health Service. Patients with a severe visual impairment are entitled to a second aid for use when the first one is out of order. (DHSS circular C291, 31.3.1980).

Hearing aids
In recent years there has been a trasformation in the range of aids available, and early in 1982 there are no fewer than nine different behind-the-ear models and three types of body-worn aids available. The behind-the-ear models consist of three series. The BE10 series (BE11, 13, 14, 15 and 16) are all moderately-powered aids, the BE13 and BE16 having forward facing microphones which may help with mobility problems. The BE30 series (BE 31 and 32) are more powerful aids and are intended for patients who are either unable to use the BE10 series or use them at maximum volume. The BE32 has a forward facing microphone. In 1982 a very high powered aid, the BE51 has just been introduced. All these aids have a T switch so that an induction loop system can be used (see page 246).

The old standard NHS aid, the Medresco body-worn aid, is gradually being withdrawn. Anyone still using a Medresco aid who has not been tested for a behind-the-ear aid should apply to the hospital which supplied the existing aid. The great advantage of the behind-the-ear aid is that the user no longer has to cope with a cord and a receiver; and body noise, so often created by the movement of the user's clothes over the receiver, is eliminated. However, a few patients will still need a body-worn aid, and so the Medresco aids are being replaced by the BW60 and BW80 series. These are for patients with severe and very severe impairment respectively and both have air conduction and bone conduction fittings.

All the NHS aids are made to DHSS specifications by commercial hearing aid manufacturers, so it is not necessarily true that a privately purchased aid must be better than a NHS one. Anyone considering buying a hearing aid would be well advised to try the appropriate NHS one first. The Royal National Institute for the Deaf issues a list of current hearing aids, which gives details of prices, and a booklet *Hearing Aids – Questions and Answers* (free on receipt of a stamped addressed envelope).

Strange as it may seem, the old-fashioned simple ear trumpet and speaking tube are often effective when all else fails, especially with the very elderly. These are still available through the NHS.

A much more sophisticated device is the Communicator, which consists of a hand-held microphone linked to a lorgnette-type amplifier. The speaker talks into the microphone in a normal voice, whilst the listener holds the lorgnette to his ear and adjusts the volume to a comfortable level. The Communicator is manufactured by *A and M Hearing Aids Ltd, 7 Kelvin Way, Crawley, Sussex RH10 2LS (tel. Crawley (0293) 26976)*.

Telephone aids
British Telecom can supply an amplifying handset or an extra earpiece which allows a deaf subscriber to listen with both ears, or which can be used by a second person to help answer the call. A new telephone aid, the inductive coupler, has recently been introduced. This can be incorporated in regular telephone handsets and the 14A amplifying handset. It works in conjunction with hearing aids which have a pick-up coil (this includes all NHS hearing aids except the old Medresco OL56). To use the coupler, the hearing aid is switched to the 'T' or 'M' position, the volume control adjusted, and the handset then is used normally. A flashing light can also be provided to work in

conjunction with the telephone bell for those who do not hear it ringing, but have a little sight. Alternatively, there is a variety of extra-loud bells available. Full details of all these aids, including rentals, can be obtained from the local telephone manager's office (sales division). Portable couplers which can be used on any standard telephone handset can be purchased on the commercial market.

Radio, television and talking book aids
The induction loop system enables any listener who has a pick-up coil incorporated in the hearing aid to listen directly through the aid to these sources of sound. Thus other members of the household are spared the annoyance of an excessively high volume level, and the listener hears more clearly and comfortably and no longer has to sit very close to the set.

Full details of how a room should be wired – an operation neither excessively complicated nor expensive – and the television and radio adapted are found in *Television/Radio Adaptors and the Loop System*, a free booklet from the Royal National Institute for the Deaf.

Talking book library members should contact their local talking book servicing volunteer who can fit the loop system, obtaining the necessary instructions from the Talking Book Library. In case of difficulty, members should contact *Mr Don Roskilly, Director of the Talking Book Library, 224 Great Portland Street, London W1N 6AA (tel. 01-388 1266)*.

There are a number of other aids available which are designed to enable listeners to hear television, radio or tape recorders more clearly. For example, a microphone can be attached to the radio or television by means of an adhesive pad and then plugged into an amplifier which rests on the arm of a chair, a device which does not need to be installed by an engineer. The user has only to plug the earphones provided into the amplifier and adjust the sound level to his preference. Full details of these aids can be obtained from the RNID.

Visual doorbells and clocks
Deaf people with residual vision may be helped by a visual doorbell with a light which flashes brightly when the bell is pressed, or by an alarm clock which rouses by a flashing light. Details can be obtained from the RNID and help with their provision, or installation, may be available from local social services departments.

Further reading
General Guidance for Hearing Aid Users is a DHSS publication available in braille from the RNIB.

Deaf-blindness
'Deaf-blindness is not the sum of two disabilities – deafness and blindness – but is instead a third and totally separate disability.' It is not known how many people in Britain suffer from this very grave disability but it is certain that the number of deaf-blind adults in the community will increase as victims of the rubella outbreaks of the 1960s reach adulthood. At present, the majority of deaf-blind adults are elderly, having developed both disabilities late in life; though a significant number of young people exhibiting Usher's or Norrey's syndrome who have been deaf from birth develop severe visual impairment or loss of sight in young adulthood.

Communication
This is the lifeline of the deaf-blind, and keeping the lines of communication open is vitally important. There are no 'right' and 'wrong' methods – whatever is acceptable to a deaf-blind individual is the method that is 'right'. Tried and trusted methods include writing messages with a thick black felt-tip pen, tracing letters using the deaf-blind person's forefinger, using the Morse code, and the widely used deaf-blind manual and 'Spartan'.

The deaf-blind manual is similar to the manual alphabet for the deaf in which the sender's fingers are used to form letters, but the letters are formed instead on the deaf-blind person's hand. Spartan is even simpler: capital letters are traced on the deaf-blind person's palm. Free leaflets illustrating both methods can be obtained from the RNIB and the Deaf-Blind Helpers' League. Practised senders and receivers can achieve relatively high speeds of communication by using the manual. Spartan, although slower, has the advantage that anybody can transmit a message without learning a new alphabet.

Deaf-blind people who read braille or Moon can use a communicator disc, issued free by the RNIB. The sighted person moves a pointer to the appropriate letter (which is shown in black print, braille and Moon), and the deaf-blind person can then read it.

A much more sophisticated device which demands good braille is the Tellatouch. This machine has a conventional typewriter keyboard on which the sighted person types the message. This is received, letter by letter, by the deaf-blind person resting his finger on a single braille cell at the back of the machine. A machine which would convert the message into a medium other than braille is still at an experimental stage. For deaf-blind people who read braille, communication by telephone is now possible. Speech can be converted into braille and received by the deaf-blind person at a terminal in his or her own home. Investigations began in 1981 to see whether demand would warrant production.

Whatever method is used, conversation is naturally difficult and makes great demands on 'speaker' and 'listener'. It is only too easy for a visitor's mind to go blank, or for everything to seem too trivial to be spelled out laboriously. Yet it is the trivial things that often give gaiety, and bring warmth and life into people's lives. It is also easy to ignore non-verbal means of communication as these tend generally to be avoided. Contact by touch is vitally important; a friendly hug or touch can mean a great deal to someone who cannot see the friendly smile or catch the concerned tone in the voice.

Aids and gadgets
Through the NHS and the RNIB a doorbell warning device is available; this consists of a ring which vibrates on a deaf-blind person's finger. It operates through an induction loop system and although when the ring vibrates on the finger there is a slight tingling sensation which could be taken to be a small electric shock, the stimulus is entirely mechanical. Understandably, no deaf-blind user is going to feel happy about this gadget until after being reassured about this. Advice on obtaining and installing this aid is available from the RNIB, but it can only be used by deaf-blind people who have a NHS body-worn aid with an induction coil.

Some deaf-blind people prefer a warning device by which strategically placed electric fans circulate air for a fixed period of time when the doorbell is pressed. Details can be obtained from the Deaf-Blind Helpers' League.

An electric tactile bedside alarm clock connected to a vibrator disc by a lead can be purchased from the RNIB. The vibrator is placed under the pillow, and is claimed to be 100 per cent effective in waking people up!

A tactile version of the very popular liquid level indicator (illustration on page 101) is being developed by the RNIB.

A red and white stick indicates that the user is deaf-blind. The RNIB supply free a wooden stick with two four-inch wide bands of red reflectorised tape attached between the handle and the tip.

There are remarkably few braille publications designed to meet the special needs of the deaf-blind. The weekly *Braille Mail* is a digest of the week's newspapers issued free by the RNIB. In Birmingham, the Elizabeth Gunn Centre (page 256) issues a daily braille digest of the previous day's radio news. The Harrogate and District Talking Newspaper produces a braille summary of local news.

Rehabilitation

Deaf-blind people can attend the RNIB's rehabilitation courses, provided the problems of communication can be solved. Rainbow Court, the headquarters of the Deaf-Blind Helpers' League at Paston Ridings, Peterborough, offers rehabilitation facilities, but no formal course is offered. Deaf-blind visitors are welcome to stay in the guest-house and, through meeting the deaf-blind residents in the League's flats, are encouraged to find means of overcoming their double handicap. Residents are ready to help a newcomer with informal instruction by means of communication, braille and Moon, and help in daily living.

Annual social rehabilitation courses for the deaf-blind are held at seaside resorts by the Northern and Southern Regional Associations for the Blind. There are sessions on communication, advice about speech therapy, with much practice of manual communication, as well as holiday outings and evening socials. Details can be obtained from the local Social Services Departments, or direct from the appropriate association. Help is almost certain to be forthcoming with meeting the fees for these courses if these might cause financial hardship.

Holiday hotels and residential homes

Deaf-blind guests, if accompanied by a guide, are generally welcome in the holiday hotels mentioned in Chapter 15. In addition, the RNIB has residential homes at Harrogate, Yorkshire, and Burnham-on-Sea, Somerset. Most residents are permanent, but guests can be accommodated for a holiday. St Anne's Holiday Home for the Blind-Deaf in Clacton-on-Sea, Essex, offers comfortable, informal and friendly accommodation at reasonable cost, with a slightly lower charge for escorts (see page 202). The guest-house at Rainbow Court is available for holidays to members of the Deaf-Blind Helpers' League, who also have a block of twelve flats for deaf-blind people wanting a permanent and independent home of their own.

Local authority services

These are provided for the deaf-blind by social services departments, generally through their schemes of services for the blind. The deaf-blind are, however, in the unfortunate position of being a very small minority requiring a highly specialised and personal service calling on skills found in workers for the deaf and workers for the blind, but rarely common to both. Some social services departments try to meet the need by providing a special guide-help service for deaf-blind people. This service was pioneered in Bristol in 1960, but has spread to other parts of the country. It involves the employment of part-time guide helps (often through the home help service) who visit the deaf-blind person regularly, and act as an escort and interpreter and help in any way needed. Some social services departments sponsor special clubs for the deaf-blind.

National Health Services

A wide range of hearing aids is now available (see page 244). Deaf-blind people who are having mobility training and would be helped by wearing a hearing aid in each ear can be issued with two aids on the recommendation of their consultant. All deaf-blind people are eligible for a spare aid (see page 244).

Speech therapy is supplied through the NHS, although speech therapists are in short supply. Conserving speech is, of course, very important, for it is only too easy for a deaf-blind person's speech to become distorted, or too soft or too loud. The family doctor or health visitor should be able to make arrangements for this service.

Voluntary Services

The Royal National Institute for the Blind employs a welfare officer whose brief is to promote services for the deaf-blind. She is available for consultation by voluntary agencies for the deaf and the blind, and by social services departments. If requested by an appropriate agency, she will visit individual deaf-blind people and advise on ways in which their needs might be met.

250

The National Deaf-Blind Helpers' League was founded in 1928. Any deaf-blind person is eligible for membership if he is registered as blind and has so little hearing that he cannot hear speech at a distance of more than a yard, even when wearing a hearing aid. Associate members undertake to take a personal interest in one deaf-blind person, and to help deaf-blind people generally whenever possible.

A quarterly magazine, *The Rainbow*, is published in braille and Moon, and extracts from it also appear quarterly in inkprint. It contains news from the various branches of the League, information of special interest to the deaf-blind, and contributions from deaf-blind members, and acts as a general forum for deaf-blind people, helping isolated members to keep in touch with people handicapped in a similar way. The League has clubs for members throughout the country.

The National Association for Deaf-Blind and Rubella Handicapped was formed originally to give support and help to parents of deaf-blind children, but its concern today is for the needs of all deaf-blind people, and especially those of the young adult (see also pages 255 and 256).

The British Usher Foundation was formed in 1980 to offer advice and help to those who suffer from Usher's syndrome, that is, a combination of hearing loss with visual loss arising from retinitis which most often attacks young adults. The Foundation hopes to raise money for research, to provide a point of contact for sufferers, and eventually establish a centre which would include accommodation for the young adult sufferer.

(For details of financial help, see pages 33–34 and 42; help for children, see pages 218–255; young adults, see pages 255–6).

Further reading
Helping People who are Deaf as well as Blind: RNIB. Free pamphet
How to Talk to a Deaf-Blind Person: National Deaf-Blind Helpers' League. Free leaflet
A Monograph on Volunteer Services for Deaf-Blind People: World Council for the Welfare of the Blind (RNIB)

Multiple sclerosis

Some people who suffer from this disease experience blurring of vision which makes reading very difficult, if not impossible. If they can no longer read ordinary print – that is print roughly the same size as that in which this book is set – they are eligible for a talking book from the Nuffield Talking Book Library for the Blind, if a consultant ophthalmologist will complete the necessary application form which they can obtain for him from the RNIB. A talking book can be enjoyed comfortably in bed by the use of pillow-phones and a remote control on/off switch, operated by gentle pressure, can be fitted. A talking book can, of course, be used also in conjunction with Possum equipment. Details can be obtained from the Talking Book Library.

People who are registered blind may find the special small radio issued by the Wireless for the Blind Fund (see page 161) easier to use than the standard Roberts set. The Multiple Sclerosis Society is at present considering issuing the *MS Bulletin* on compact cassette to visually handicapped members and would welcome enquiries. Some people who are unable to walk have been able to make use of a sonic device fitted into their wheelchairs (see page 131).

Amputees

Fortunately it is uncommon in peacetime to meet the dual handicap of visual loss and loss of a limb. St Dunstan's have, however, a wide and long experience of the problems faced by blind people who have lost the use of a limb, and are only too willing to pass on the benefit of their experience to the civilian visually handicapped. They are always willing to give details of the aids they have designed over the years, and which have been proved to be effective. A series of leaflets shows photographs of these, and can be obtained from St Dunstan's. Details of their semi-automatic cassette changer for talking book machines are given below.

People with restricted movement

Many visually handicapped people, being elderly, come into this category. Aids to help cope with problems such as getting into and out of the bath, out of a chair, off the toilet and climbing stairs are available. The range is vast. People need to study what is available for their particular handicap and select those aids that also meet, or can be modified to meet, their visual needs. Few people have the facilities to do this for themselves, but advice on, and assessment for, appropriate aids, should be available from social services departments and the daily living departments (occupational therapy departments) in hospitals. Day hospitals, day centres or rehabilitation centres are other possible sources of help. The Disabled Living Foundation has a permanent display of such aids on show and similar centres exist in Birmingham, Leicester, Liverpool, Manchester and Newcastle. (The addresses for these centres are given at the beginning of *Useful Addresses*, page 271.)

Visually handicapped people with impaired hands who have difficulty using the controls on their talking book can have the switches modified. A bar can be fitted to the on/off switch, for example, so that the machine can be switched on and off by pushing the bar with the back of the hand. The playback machine can also be fitted with a semi-automatic cassette changer, operated by the forearm, which accurately locates the cassette on the reproducer, withdraws it, and turns the cassette over preparatory to playing the next track. Full details can be obtained from the Talking Book Library. People who find it difficult to fit and remove the mains plug from its socket might find the Extracta plug handle (Newton Aids Ltd.) helpful. This handle fits over the standard Crabtree three-pin plug. It can easily be removed for use elsewhere.

The multi-handicapped
At both ends of the age range, it is now increasingly rare to find anyone whose sole handicap is visual impairment. The phrase 'multi-handicap' is, however, generally used in the context of the needs of children and adults rather than the elderly, whose needs are discussed in Chapter 18. It implies a mix of disability, in which visual, physical and mental handicaps often all play a part.

Services for this group have always been and still are notable mainly for their scarcity, although in recent years considerably more attention has been focused on them. The extension of the 1944 Education Act to cover children who previously had been classified as ineducable, led to an increasing identification of the multi-handicapped and, from 1970, the opening of units for them in various parts of the country, although there is still little specialist 'blind' provision. Indeed, in 1980, it was pointed out in a House of Lords debate that, outside the hospital service, there existed only 200 special places.

The Southern and Western Regional Association for the Blind has set up, and is sponsoring, a Committee on the Multi-Handicapped Blind to investigate the needs of multi-handicapped blind people and to identify ways of meeting those needs. The Committee is willing to offer advice and help, where possible, and to collaborate with individuals or groups having similar aims in respect of this population. They are preparing a directory of services for the visually and mentally handicapped for circulation to NHS establishments for the mentally handicapped; this will be available at a small charge to other interested people.

Two organisations serving the interests of the mentally handicapped also have a concern for those who suffer from visual impairment as well. The British Institute of Mental Handicap specialises in training courses and informative literature. Their quarterly publication, *Apex*, is a valuable source of information and often carries articles concerning visual handicaps.

The Association of Professions for the Mentally Handicapped is a multi-disciplinary organisation which has numerous local branches throughout the country where regular meetings are held. Membership is open to parents, relatives and other interested people as well as to professionals. *Information Sheet* is a recently introduced and valuable source of practical information and ideas regarding ways of teaching mentally and visually handicapped children. It is produced by a group of special education teachers and can be obtained by sending a stamped addressed envelope to *David Bethell, Child Guidance Centre, Little Street West, Walsall WS2 8EN*.

An excellent free booklet *Guidelines for Teachers and Parents of Visually Handicapped Children with Additional Handicaps* is issued by the RNIB. Any parent whose child attends a centre not specifically for the blind should make sure that a copy reaches the staff who have day-to-day contact with his child.

Services

Much of the information in Chapters 16 and 17 is relevant to the needs of multi-handicapped children. The RNIB Education Advisory Service, for example, can provide visiting advisers, some of whom specialise in the education of mentally handicapped or deaf-blind children. Listed below, however, are the main centres which aim to cater especially for them.

Education

All special schools for the visually handicapped and all Sunshine Homes admit children with additional handicaps. One primary school (Rushton Hall, Kettering) and one secondary school (Condover Hall, near Shrewsbury) provide expressly for blind children with additional handicaps. Condover Hall also has a special department (Pathways) for children between five and seventeen years with communication problems involving poor sight and poor hearing. In addition a few special units for children with defects of sight and hearing are attached to special or ordinary schools in various parts of the country.

The National Centre for Deaf-Blind Children and their families, was opened in 1980 to meet the needs of 'rubella' children. These children are born handicapped because their mother suffered from German measles in pregnancy. Such children are likely to suffer sight defects, deafness, mental handicap or heart lesions, and often have a combination of all or three of these conditions. The Centre contains a mother and baby unit for parents of very young deaf-blind children, a teaching unit for children between three and eleven years, short stay facilities at weekends or during school holidays and a resource centre of books, play and teaching equipment. Courses are also arranged for parents, relatives and professionals. The address is *86 Cleveland Road, Ealing, London W13 (tel. 01-991 0513).*

The Royal School for Deaf Children, Margate, has established a special education unit for hearing-impaired children with additional handicaps such as blindness, specific learning difficulties and physical handicaps, while the Royal National Institute for the Deaf is developing a teaching and residential facility at Poole Mead in Bath, for deaf-blind young people and adults with additional handicaps.

Residential and training facilities are also available within the NHS for more severely mentally handicapped children. These include the Ellen Terry Home in Reigate, the Mary Sheridan Unit at Borocourt Hospital in Berkshire and the facility at Lea Castle Hospital, Kidderminster. Details of all these resources can be obtained from the RNIB Education Department.

Further education/vocational assessment

Many multi-handicapped school-leavers need time to mature and an opportunity to widen their experience of life before they are ready to cope with the rough and tumble of the world beyond the residential centres where they may have spent most of their lives.

The Queen Alexandra College, Birmingham, offers a special maturation course for this group, working closely with the Elizabeth Gunn Centre see below.

Greenside, Liverpool (The Catholic Blind Institute) offers a two-year course for multi-handicapped adolescent girls and aims by intensive care, the provision of new opportunities and the chance to take part in all the sighted activities of a big city, to enable them to move on to a vocational assessment centre or further training and eventually into open employment.

The Manor House, Market Deeping (The National Association for the Deaf-Blind and Rubella Handicapped) has similar aims and is a residential hostel, with associated sheltered workshop, catering for the needs of deaf-blind school-leavers with additional handicaps.

Another centre for the deaf-blind, Poole Mead, Bath (Royal National Institute for the Deaf) is nearing completion in 1981. Yet there is still a great shortage of specialist accommodation for multi-handicapped school-leavers who, for one reason or another, cannot live at home. A new centre, possibly in the north-east, is under discussion in 1981. Details of the current situation can be obtained from the RNIB Education Department. They are also ready to advise on suitable placements and when appropriate will refer enquirers to the After-Care Officer, Condover Hall, who has a wide experience in this field.

Employment

It has to be recognised that some multi-handicapped young people, even with the best of training, are so seriously handicapped that employment, even in the sheltered schemes described on page 51, is not a realistic goal. For those living at home, attendance at the local Adult Training Centre or a day centre for the physically handicapped may be satisfactory placements. Local social services departments can give details and arrange trial visits. The Elizabeth Gunn Centre (Birmingham Royal Institution for the Blind) is probably unique in that it is a day centre specifically for blind people with additional handicaps. It caters for those living in the Birmingham area, but has a small residential unit, 'Oakwood', which provides bed-sitting room accommodation. All training and day centres provide simple paid work and although earnings are often at a 'pocket-money' level, they can be a welcome addition to state benefits.

Residential centres

Apart from Manor House and Oakwood, only two other specialist residential establishments cater for severely handicapped blind and partially sighted young people.

The Royal School for the Blind, Leatherhead, is by far the largest, with 150 residents. It is in the process of a massive modernisation scheme which should be completed in 1984. The present Victorian buildings are being transformed into five self-contained hostels with bed-sitting room accommodation, and some flats for married couples. The Royal School accepts suitable applicants who may suffer from one or a combination of additional handicaps, and aims to offer an environment which gives warmth, care, support and stimulation, whilst at the same time developing realistic independence.

The Wilberforce Home, York, is a much smaller purpose-built home catering for blind people between the ages of sixteen and thirty-five years on admission who have a serious physical handicap that prevents them from working. Applications for Leatherhead and York should be made through the social services department in the applicant's home area. Payment of fees is as described on page 61.

It is sadly true, however, that young people who cannot be placed in specialised residential facilities for the visually and mentally handicapped, may drift into long-term residence in hospitals unless they are reasonably independent in daily living skills. An encouraging new development aimed to prevent this drift is the founding of the Peppard Trust by professional staff associated with the Mary Sheridan Unit (page 255). The Trust was set up to allow work to continue with the deaf-blind multiply disabled severely educationally subnormal children who become too old for the Mary Sheridan Unit and who would, otherwise, become institutionalised long-term residents of hospitals for the mentally handicapped. The Trust's aim is to combine the provision of a national short-stay diagnostic and advisory facility with long-stay training services when appropriate, research into the development of social and physical skills and the eventual provision for the accommodation and training of parents. A few of the large hospitals for the mentally handicapped are also looking for ways to set up residential and occupational facilities which are better suited to the needs of their blind residents.

Staff training

Encouraging staff to develop appropriate teaching and care skills is vital to the future interests of the visually and mentally handicapped in long-stay hospitals. Both the Southern and Western Regional Association for the Blind and the British Institute of Mental Handicap are prepared to provide travelling workshops of teachers who will visit local centres and present talks and training courses to interested staff in hospitals. The SWRAB service is provided free of charge. The National Association of Deaf-Blind and Rubella Handicapped are willing to offer a similar service to staff working with deaf-blind people according to need. The Department of Special Education at the University of Birmingham offers professional training for teachers with respect to the needs of visual and mental handicaps in children. The department frequently accepts student teachers from ESN(S) schools.

★ *If you have to take two or more different kinds of medicines and want to be sure not to mix them up, put each box of pills or bottle of medicine into an easily distinguishable larger container, such as an empty margarine carton or a tea caddy. It is important to store medicines in the container in which they were originally dispensed.*
(Roger Hitchens, Bristol)

★ *Following an eye operation, I was told to avoid looking down and eating meals was a problem. To avoid kneeling at the dinner table I had the idea of putting my plate on top of a three tier cake tin which brought it up to my eye level!*
(Anne Holden, Newcastle)

How to help

There is a lot of goodwill towards blind people expressed by the population generally but many people who are keen to 'do something to help the blind' are uncertain how to translate their good intentions into positive and helpful action. For any individual who would like to help, but is uncertain where to begin, the best start would be to contact either the local social services department, or the local voluntary society for the blind, who are most likely to know what is needed in their own locality. Friendly sighted helpers at clubs for the blind, particularly those who can help with transport, are likely to be needed in most locations. The addresses of all local agencies for the blind are given in the 'Directory of Agencies for the Blind' published by the RNIB. However it is not only through 'blind' organisations that sighted people can help: most people think of reading as being the obvious service that a sighted friend can give to a blind person, but it is probably true to say that almost any talent can be put to use to help. The enthusiastic photographer might be able to link up with a partially sighted person who, with the aid of a suitable camera and enlargements, can actually manage to see in a photograph what he or she cannot see in ordinary life. An avid cyclist might care to be steersman on a tandem for a blind child or adult who could not otherwise enjoy cycling. Someone who has a basic knowledge of music can be an enormous help to poorly sighted musicians as large print music is virtually non-existent, and scores have to be copied by hand. In recent years yachting has become a popular sport among many blind people, and experienced yachtsmen who would be prepared to let a blind person crew are always in demand. There is an amazing variety of activities with which volunteers of all ages can help blind people in various parts of Britain. Pottery, drama, gardening, bell-ringing, dancing and rambling are just a few of the activities set up by enthusiastic volunteers. In fact one could probably say that there is hardly any leisure activity which some blind person somewhere hasn't tackled – and often it has been made possible by a sighted expert's help.

There is no shortage of people who feel that they would like to read to the blind; but – while many blind people *do* need readers – it may well be that the expectations of the volunteer reader and the recipient are widely different. The inexperienced volunteer frequently assumes that it will involve reading aloud from a novel, thriller or other entertaining book; but the actual needs of a blind person are for someone who would read more prosaic things like the details of the telephone bill, the runners at the day's races or the instruction leaflet for a piece of household equipment, several times over if necessary. As with all volunteer services it is crucial that someone who offers help not only ensures that what is being given is what is actually needed, but also is what he or she is really able to do well. A volunteer reader who has an unfulfilled urge to read novels aloud, may not get much satisfaction out of reading someone's cooker manual; but for those with good reading voices there may be scope for their services in one of the tape reading services which have been set up in recent years. These services will put on to tape any printed material requested by a blind person – whether it's a knitting pattern, cookery recipes or the details of an insurance policy, and all services depend on volunteers who are capable of making recordings at home on their own equipment. (See Chapter 13, *Pleasures of listening*, for details). For those who feel they can help on an individual basis there are a number of ways in which would-be readers can be linked up to someone who would welcome their help. Local voluntary societies or social service departments may be able to match individual readers with a blind person requiring help in their own neighbourhood. Alternatively any would-be reader who makes himself known to the Matron of a local residential home for the elderly, or contacts the sister-in-charge of the geriatric ward in the local hospital is almost sure to find plenty of people who would be delighted to make use of his services.

It is worth noting that it is not only the able-bodied who can help. One particularly felicitous arrangement which a blind lady in Cambridge enjoyed for several years was with a housebound disabled neighbour whom she visited once a week in order to have the local paper read to her. The other, ever-growing, organisation which is glad of readers, who are prepared to commit themselves on a regular basis, is the Talking Newspaper Association. At the time of writing there are over 300 local talking newspapers, which in cassette form reproduce an edited version of the local newspaper. The production of these taped newspapers is labour-intensive; apart from people who can read the news, volunteers are needed to help with the recording and editing of the tapes, and even those with no reading abilities or technical skill can help to pack up and distribute the finished product. In some areas the weekly visit from a volunteer worker from the Talking Newspaper is a highlight and the visit can in fact be an opportunity – if it seems appropriate – for the visitor to offer help in other ways as well. Fitting an electrical plug is less than five minutes' effort for most sighted people, but blind people have sometimes waited for weeks before they had a visitor whom they could ask to help with something as simple.

For people who enjoy simple technical tasks, there is always a need for volunteers to service the radio sets issued by the Wireless for the Blind Fund. The Fund is keen to recruit people who will take on the responsibility of looking after the radios of blind people in a particular locality – so that they can help blind people to use the equipment and visit them on request if the machine gives any trouble. A similar function is needed for the Talking Book Service. Volunteers are needed initially to show blind people how to work the machines, and to service them when necessary. This does not call for any high degree of electronic competence – according to the Director of the Talking Book Service, 'all you need is someone who knows what to do with a screwdriver'.

But it is not necessary to have a special skill to help a blind person – sparing time to take a blind person for a walk in the park or a drive down to the shops is very much appreciated particularly by the more elderly blind. Help with transport – whether for individual journeys to do shopping or visit a friend, or to keep an appointment with the doctor – is probably the single most important type of help needed by blind people, particularly those living in areas not well served by public transport. But even where buses exist, older blind people may find it such a strain to travel alone on public transport that they may opt to stay at home.

One group of blind people who are often very cut off from the community are the residents in homes for the elderly. When about thirty matrons of such homes were asked by *In Touch* about ways in which volunteers could contribute, almost all said that they needed help for taking residents out. Walks in the fresh air, or rides in a car, are treats that hard-pressed staff have not got the means to organise. A number of matrons said also that although they had young volunteers offering to help, these were not really so satisfactory as older people who would be more sensitive to the needs of elderly people and better able to communicate with them. Several matrons mentioned wistfully that it might be nice to find a local person who could play some of the old tunes on the piano to entertain their residents!

Simple mending is another chore which often gets left undone in

Homes for the Elderly, as well as by individual blind people living in their own homes; a sighted friend who will sew on buttons, do simple repairs, straighten a hem or let out a waistband would be a boon to many blind people. In one area, some retired nuns undertook all the mending for the local blind people. ,

But in addition to the help that can be given by individuals there has, in the last decade, been quite a lot of change in the services provided by local voluntary societies. In the past many had contented themselves (and their clients) with annual outings, Christmas gifts and entertainments or financial help with special needs. But in the wake of the Seebohm reorganisation of the social services, many voluntary societies recognised that with the disappearance of the specialist (Home) teacher, there was often no one in the local social service department with special skills or knowledge related to the needs of people with little or no sight. Effectively it was often the volunteer in a given locality who had become the 'specialist' in blind welfare. Now, in 1981 – after more than ten years of generic social services – in some areas the voluntary society has become a resource from which local blind people can get help and information.

Quite a number of voluntary societies produce booklets giving information on aids and services available locally and nationally. The booklets are generally aimed at the newly-blind and their relatives; some are in large print to help the partially sighted. In Inverness the local society distributes its pamphlet through eye clinics so that patients can get some basic information without having first to be visited by a social worker. Other societies sometimes make use of local talking newspapers or radio stations to disseminate information. But an increasing number of voluntary societies are also taking on the task of providing a resource centre where a variety of aids and equipment are on permanent display. One of the pioneers in this field was the Surrey Voluntary Association, which has not only got together information about equipment of use to the blind, but bulk buys equipment – such as talking clocks – which are otherwise only available from commercial sources and sells them at a subsidised rate to local blind people. In Bristol, the local society has its own Home for the Elderly, within which it has equipped a 'show flat' with every kind of aid and appliance that might be of use in a blind person's home, so that local people can come and try them out in a realistic setting.

As more people become aware of the help that can be given to make the best use of limited vision, there is a growing interest in low vision aids. This is an area in which blind people find it difficult to get advice from experts unless they are fortunate enough to be referred to low vision aid clinics, which invariably have long waiting lists. Not all opticians carry a wide range of magnifiers, and it is not easy for someone with limited vision to get to see the various types of low vision aids that are available. To try and overcome these problems both the Partially Sighted Society and the Disabled Living Foundation have put together selections of magnifiers for the benefit of anyone concerned with the care or rehabilitation of blind people. The Partially Sighted Society kit, which costs £120, has samples of the basic types of magnifier; these can either be demonstrated at club meetings or taken round to homes, hospitals or day centres. Thus visually handicapped people get a chance to see a wider range of aids than might be available in a local shop. At least one society (Berkshire) arranges for a local ophthalmologist to visit its clubs regularly to talk about low vision aids. The Disabled Living Foundation has a much more comprehensive selection of all kinds of low vision aids which is available for hire in their 'flying suitcase' as a resource to enable professionals to update their knowledge of low vision aids.

A number of societies have purchased a closed-circuit television set so that local people can come in to read their letters or any other printed material. The purchase of such extremely expensive equipment for use by a large number of blind people means that in principle it is available to people who would never be able to afford to buy one for themselves: but it has to be stated that a number of societies that had bought sets told *In Touch* that they had been disappointed that relatively little use had been made of them. It is not clear why this should be. Some societies feel that it is difficult for elderly blind people to get used to the equipment – or that they may simply find it a strain, and prefer to have their letters read to them. Perhaps also the siting of the equipment may influence its use – not everyone wants to read their private letters on an enlarged screen in a busy office where quite a number of people could easily see the enlarged letters – even if they did not want to pry!

Elsewhere voluntary societies have used their funds to build accommodation for blind people. In Norwich the local society has built a block of flats, supervised by a warden, to serve as sheltered accommodation for elderly, active blind people. Henshaws Society for the Blind have added to their residential home in Rhyl a special care centre, which is a half-way house to accommodate people who need more care than can be provided in a residential home.

But it does not need vast capital expenditure to help a blind person with housing. It is often difficult for a blind person to take up a job in a strange city because landlords are reluctant to rent accommodation to them. So a friendly landlady who is prepared to take in a blind man – or woman – who needs no special care may mean that this person is able to work – as often it is not possible for a blind person to find a job in his own home town.

Whatever voluntary societies can provide by way of amenities paid for from their funds, in the end their main resource is people – and the disappearance of the home teacher who was a regular and welcome visitor to the homes of many blind people has left a gap which many voluntary societies are now attempting to fill. A number of societies have set up specific visiting services, recruiting and training their volunteers. Devon have for some time run their 'match a visitor' scheme, in which each blind person is paired with a specially trained volunteer with whom they have as many interests as possible in common. Hampshire have started a comprehensive visiting and monitoring service, to mitigate some of the effects of the cutback in local authority spending which meant that many blind people never saw a social worker unless they were in a 'crisis situation'. But even in more prosperous times, the generally accepted social work interpretation of 'crisis' does not, unfortunately, include the trauma of sight loss – so that after the initial post-registration visit most blind people would not be seen again by a social worker, unless some other mishap befell them.

In addition to visiting and befriending the average elderly blind person, there is also a tremendous need for dedicated people who can undertake the task of learning to communicate with people who have the double disadvantage of hearing and sight loss. The National Deaf-Blind Helpers League would always be very happy to advise would-be helpers. And although braille is of use to only a relatively small proportion of blind people, there is a steady demand for braille transcribers. To learn braille to a sufficiently high standard by correspondence course may take up to a year but a number of retired people as well as younger people with time to spare have found it a fascinating and rewarding pursuit. Details of training schemes can be obtained from the RNIB or any of the braille transcription services listed on pages 145/6.

But perhaps the most important lesson for any would-be volunteer to learn is to check whether the proposed help is really wanted. There are endless tales of blind people who have been taken to the other side of a road they did not want to cross! Even more classic as a misconceived gesture of goodwill is the scented garden planted in a park. Most blind people are more than happy to enjoy the scent of flowers in parks or gardens intended for the general public, but they do not want to be segregated to sniff the flowers! Unfortunately, while well-meaning people will spend time and energy in making a scented garden, it is rare for someone who takes the trouble to design and lay out these gardens to ensure that there will always be an escort to get blind visitors safely to the garden.

Consultations with local blind people about any new project dreamed up by volunteers should be automatic: it was interesting to see in a survey carried out in 1978 by Enid Dance, a blind lady in Guildford, among local blind people that the service most wanted was help with bulk buying of non-perishable household goods (for example, detergents and toilet rolls), but not one of over seventy local societies around the country contacted by *In Touch* to see what services they provided, mentioned any bulk-buying scheme.

Often it may be just a very small gesture which may make all the difference. In one hospital which had a lot of elderly patients with limited vision, the arrival of a volunteer once or twice a week to polish their glasses effected a dramatic improvement in the old ladies' eyesight. One does not always have to spend £1,000 to help a visually handicapped person make the most of their remaining sight!

21 Finding other ways

Rehabilitation includes the process of finding other ways. An eighty-year-old who appeared on the *In Touch* programme – she had been blind for less than two years – brushed aside all her difficulties by saying: 'After all, it's your hands that do the work, your eyes only tell you where to put them.' You are halfway to success in anything you tackle once you acquire the art of making it sound much easier than it really is.

There is a pleasant myth, put about by well-meaning sighted people, that the blind are more courageous, more gifted and more cheerful than the rest of humanity. Most of us would like to believe that we have most of these qualities most of the time, but we know, when we are honest with ourselves, that sometimes we are chicken-hearted, sometimes we are ham-fisted and sometimes we are down in the dumps. But this is because we are people, not because we are blind. There is no such thing as a composite 'image of the blind' because blind people are different from each other in the same way as athletes are different from each other, or soldiers, or mountaineers, in the same way as finger-prints are different. But in at least one aspect of blindness we are all united. We want to earn for ourselves a place at the conference table, a stake in the affairs of men, we want to belong to the immediate community in which we live and to the world-wide community, the brotherhood of man. It is on this basis that blind people use *In Touch*, not merely to talk to each other but to talk to all people. We begin from the premise that sensible, unselfconscious personal relationships spring from better understanding.

The expression 'the blind leading the blind' is usually taken to mean that two people, instead of one, are getting nowhere fast. In certain circumstances, being blind is the best qualification one can have for leading another blind person. It was said by one blind man who appeared on the programme that it was the wives and husbands of newly-blind people who really needed rehabilitation. Certainly, in some respects, the difficulties are as great for the partner as they are for the person who has become blind. I don't think blind people want the world turned upside-down for their benefit; their aim is to fit into a normal environment. But a blind person's wife or husband can be a tremendous help in many small ways.

I recall an interview with Tom Drake, Principal of the RNIB

Rehabilitation Centre at Torquay, who brought to the studio twenty-five years of experience in dealing with newly-blind people and their families. He stressed the importance of not moving things. A blind person depends very much on being able to put his hand immediately on something he wants, in the very place where he last put it down. If he had not been methodical before he lost his sight, he had better start learning to be methodical now! It may take a blind man a very long time to find an ashtray if it is moved one foot away from its usual position. This does not imply that blind people are singularly helpless, and a family does not need to reorient itself completely in order to cope with a blind parent. But it can undermine the confidence of a newly-blind person when things are never in the same place twice. It is helpful not to place ornaments on the corners of sideboards and shelves. And if you place a cup of tea in front of someone who cannot see, just in case you have been very quiet about it, tell him that it's there. Don't wait until he knocks it over.

Tom Drake, I remember, made another point which is possibly more important than any of this. When a husband and father loses his sight – and this applies with equal cogency to a wife and mother – don't try to shield either of them from the day-to-day cares of the family; don't cut them out of family conferences and concerns. More than ever before, they need to feel that they have a part to play. They don't want to be set aside. It's a natural tendency for people to say 'Don't worry your father, he has enough on his plate.' Of course he wants to be worried, when worrying means having a share in the normal cares of the family.

To do things for youself in your own way and in your own time, to stand on your own feet, to find your level of independence and achievement – these are the things which bring confidence and self-respect. But blind people are not normally dropped off in the middle of the Sahara Desert and expected to find their way home again. It is normal for everyone, blind or sighted, to enjoy some degree of dependence on others. Whenever I am caught up in a discussion on mobility, the relative merits of the long cane, the short cane, the guide dog, the electronic devices, I recall the blind man who said to me, no doubt with a twinkle in his eye: 'Of course, the best mobility aid which has ever been invented is a sighted wife.'

What are the practical ways in which other members of the family can help a newly-blind person? One of the most important things, like Hamlet's advice to the players, is to 'use all gently', that is, not to make a great business of reorganising the household for the benefit of its blind member. Getting a new slant on everyday things should come naturally. There is no sense in saying to a blind person: 'Would you like one of these?' unless you tell him what they are. It's no good nodding your head in agreement, because he can't hear it rattle unless there is something loose inside! So there is some quality of adaptation demanded in the family of a blind man or woman but it is not necessary to make heavy weather of it. There is no harm in making life easier for someone, whether handicapped or not. There is no harm in humanising the environment.

It is not possible to lay down a rigid set of rules on how to live with a blind person, because blind people, like all the rest of the world, have different skills – some will be expert at managing nearly everything for themselves, others will need a helping hand from time to time. In most cases, it is a matter of being able to offer unobtrusive help when it is needed. There is a little give and take required, but this is true of all human relationships. As for help being proffered when it is not really necessary, I can best illustrate what I mean by giving an example, one which has the merit of being culled from real life.

About twenty years ago, before I lost my sight, I was one day standing beside my car in the office car park, screwdriver in hand, about to dive under the bonnet. I was cocking my ear, listening to the engine ticking over. I leaned forward purposefully, screwdriver at the ready. At this moment, a colleague joined me and asked what was wrong. 'Nothing really,' I replied, 'I'm adjusting the slow running.' He bent over with me. 'It *is* running a bit fast,' he commented and it was plain that his fingers were twitching as he watched me apply the screwdriver. I solemnly handed him the screwdriver and he calmly continued the work which I had started. After a few moments 'I don't think you'll get it any better than that,' he said as he returned the screwdriver to me. 'Thank you,' I said. I'm sure this was no great hardship for me to let him do the job, especially as he was suffering so much watching me do it, but it does demonstrate that it is not only blind people who are at the mercy, so to speak, of those who are determined to help.

It's easy to say and hard to do, but the best thing that can happen to a blind person in his own home is for the family to take it in their stride, to behave naturally, to make things easier whenever and wherever they can, without seeming to do so and without making a burden of it. Above all, if he is trying to do it for himself, don't take the screwdriver away from him, don't stand there twitching.

There is not a formidable list of don'ts but an important one is not to do things for him which he is perfectly capable of doing for himself. In hotels, on railway stations, and in other places, I have often been shown where the telephone is. I wish I had a pound for every time a kindly stranger has offered to dial the number for me!

It is a very comforting thing that people are keen to help but sometimes, human nature being what it is, they tend to overdo it. This is not without its comic side. I have noticed that when I take a walk along estate roads with my guide-dog and, as occasionally happens, my attention has wandered and I am not sure where I am, I wait for someone to pass and ask, for example, 'Is this Furzehill Road?' Every time I've asked this question, the answer has been the same. 'Where do you want to go?' The simple truth is I know where I want to go. What I'm asking is 'Where am I now?' But this is no excuse for being brusque with a helpful stranger.

What I like best of all is for people to be themselves and not to put on something special because they are talking to a blind man. We are all members of the same club – it's called 'the human race' – and when we meet, there is one thing which every one of us is capable of. It comes to my mind now in an adaptation of a familiar nursery rhyme.

This is the gulf between people.

This is the bridge that spans the gulf between people.

This is the hand that builds the bridge that spans the gulf between people.

In my case, there is an emphasis on the hand and I'll tell you why. One of the questions I am frequently asked is this: 'Having lost your sight in adult life, what do you miss most?' I always find this difficult to answer because I seldom think about the things I miss. This is not nobility of character or anything of that kind. It is simply because there isn't time to worry about the things I miss while I'm so fully occupied with the things I can hit. But if I thought long and hard, I believe that not being able to catch your eye would come high on the list. This is often the first and possibly the most sensitive contact between people. I look at you and catch your eye, we exchange a glance. That's the reason for the emphasis, in my case, on the *hand* that builds the bridge.

Occasionally, when someone speaks to me, he will put his hand lightly on my sleeve, to make contact, a substitute for catching my eye. I consider this the friendliest of gestures. Often, a blind person is addressed through his companion. 'Does he take sugar?' 'Would he like to sit here?'

I suppose that's the advantage of travelling with a guide dog for companion and escort. Nobody says to the dog: 'Would your master like a cup of tea?' It's perfectly understandable that a blind person should be addressed indirectly, simply because the speaker cannot catch his eye. But he can touch him on the sleeve, he can make personal and intimate contact with him, just as a momentous and poignant contact was made, two thousand years ago, by someone touching the hem of the Master's robe.

David Scott Blackhall

Useful addresses

The addresses listed below are of organisations or individuals which are referred to frequently in the book and are given here in alphabetical order for easy reference. It is not a comprehensive list of organisations of and for the blind. This can be found in the Directory of Agencies for the Blind, published by the Royal National Institute for the Blind.

The *Aids Centres* have been set up in various centres to help disabled people, their families and those concerned with their care. They are a helpful source of advice on a wide range of aids and services, including these of help to the visually handicapped. The Disabled Living Foundation in London employs an ophthalmic optician on a part-time basis to deal with letters and telephone enquiries from visually handicapped people. Most of the aids centres prefer people to phone for an appointment before visiting.

Aids Centres

BIRMINGHAM:
Disabled Living Centre, 84 Suffolk Street, Birmingham B1 1TA (021-643 0980)

EDINBURGH:
South Lothian Aids, Distribution and Exhibition Centre, Astley Ainsley Hospital, Grange Loan, Edinburgh EH9 2HL (031-447 9200)

GLASGOW:
Aids, Advice, Information and Resource Centre, 26 Florence Street, Glasgow (041-429 2878)

LEEDS:
The Willaim Merritt Aids Centre, St. Mary's Hospital, Greenhill Road, Leeds LS12 3QE (Leeds (0532) 793140)

LEICESTER:
Medical Aids Department, 76 Clarendon Park Road, Leicester LE2 3AD (Leicester (0533) 700747/8)

LIVERPOOL:
Merseyside Aids Centre, Youens Way, East Prescot Road, Liverpool L14 2EP (051-228 9221)

LONDON:
Disabled Living Foundation, 346 Kensington High Street, London W14 8NS (01-602 2491)

NEWCASTLE-UPON-TYNE:
Aids Centre and Information Service, MEA House, Ellison Place, Newcastle-upon-Tyne NE1 8XS (Newcastle-upon-Tyne (0632) 323617)

ROTHERHAM:
General Library, Rotherham District General Hospital, Moorgate Road, Rotherham, S. Yorkshire S60 2UD (Rotherham (0709) 62222 Ext. 525)

SOUTHAMPTON:
The Aids Centre, Southampton General Hospital, Shirley, Southampton (0703) 777222 Ext. 3414)

STOCKPORT:
Aids and Assessment Unit, Stepping Hill Hospital, Stockport, Greater Manchester (061-483 1010 Ext. 207)

WAKEFIELD:
National Demonstration Centre, Pinderfields General Hospital, Aberford Road, Wakefield, Yorkshire (Wakefield (0924) 75217 Ext. 2510)

Advice Service for Blind Parents and Blind Children
see Parents Telephone Service

Advisory Centre for Education, 18 Victoria Park Square, London E2 9PB (01-980 4596)

Age Concern, Bernard Sunley House, 60 Pitcairn Road, Mitcham, Surrey CR4 3LL (01-640 5431)

American Foundation for the Blind, 15 West 16th Street, New York, NY 10011 USA (212) 620 2000

Association for the Education and Welfare of the Visually Handicapped, Hon. Sec. Mrs S. Clamp, Lickey Grange School, Old Birmingham Road, Bromsgrove, Herford and Worcester (021-445 1066)

Association of Blind and Partially Sighted Teachers & Students, BM Box 6727 London WC1V 6XX. Hon. Sec. Mrs F. White, (Northampton (0604) 411778)

Association of Blind Chartered Physiotherapists, 206 Great Portland Street, London W1N 6AA (01-387 1550)

Association of Blind Piano Tuners. Secretary: Mrs D.E. Milsted c/o R.N.I.B. 224 Great Portland Street, London W1N 6AA (01-388 1266)

Association of Professions for the Mentally Handicapped, 126 Albert Street, London NW1 7NF (01-267 6111)

Association of Visually Handicapped Office Workers, Hon. Sec. Miss E. Siekmann, 14 Verulam House, Hammersmith Grove, London W6 (01-749 1372 evenings)

Association of Visually Handicapped Telephonists, Chairman: Mr D. Lidstone, 36 Tintagel House, Salisbury Road, Edmonton N9 9TS (01-803 9095 evenings)

Birmingham Royal Institution for the Blind, Queen Alexandra Technical College, 49 Court Oak Raod, Harborne, Birmingham B17 9TG (021-427 2248)

British Association for Sporting and Recreational Activities of the Blind, c/o Sports and Recreation Officer, R.N.I.B. 224/6/8 Great Portland Street, London W1N 6AA (01-388 1266)

British Computer Association of the Blind, BCM, Box 950, London WC1N 3XX. Hon.Sec. Gerald Neal, (Guildford (0483) 68121 Ext. 373)

British Diabetic Association, 10 Queen Anne Street, London W1M 0BD (01-323 1531)

British Institute of Mental Handicap, Wolverhampton Road, Kidderminster, Worcestershire DY10 3PP (Kidderminster (0562) 850251)

Blind Mobility Research Unit, Department of Psychology, University of Nottingham, University Park, Nottingham NG7 2RD (Nottingham (0602) 56101 Ext. 3187)

British Red Cross, 9 Grosvenor Crescent, London SW1X 7EJ (01-235 5454)

British Retinitis Pigmentosa Society, Hon.Sec. Mrs L.M. Drummond-Walker, 24 Palmer Close, Redhill, Surrey RH1 4BX (Redhill (0737) 61937)

British Talking Book Service for the Blind, Mount Pleasant, Alperton, Wembley, Middlesex HA0 1RR (01-903 6666)

British Wireless for the Blind Fund, 226 Great Portland Street, London W1N 6AA (01-388 1266)

Calibre, Aylesbury, Buckinghamshire HP20 1HU (Aylesbury (0296) 32339)

Catholic Blind Institute, Christopher Grange, Youens Way, East Prescot Road, Liverpool L14 2EW (051-220 2525)

Cedric Chivers, 93-100 Locksbrook Road, Bath BA1 3EN (Bath (0225) 316872)

Circle of Guide Dog Owners, c/o Miss A. Yates, Oak Tree Cottage, Watery Lane, Corley Moor, Coventry, Warwick CV7 4AJ (Fillongley (0676) 40951)

Clerics Group, Committee Secretary, c/o RNIB, 224 Great Portland Street, London W1N 6AA (01-388 1266) ·

Counsel and Care for the Elderly (Elderly Invalids' Fund), 131 Middlesex Street, London E1 7JF (01-621 1624)

Department of Health and Social Security, Leaflets Unit, PO Box 21, Stanmore, Middlesex HA7 1AY

Department of Special Education, University of Birmingham, Ring Road North, Birmingham B15 2TT (Birmingham (021) 472 1301 Ext. 3387)

Deutsche Blindenstudienanstalt, D.3550 Marburg 1, Am Schlag 8, Federal Republic of Germany (Tel. (6421) 67053)

Disability Alliance, 21 Star Street, London W2 1QB (01-402 7026)

Disablement Income Group, Attlee House, Toynbee Hall, 28 Commercial Street, London E1 6LR (01-247 2128)

Electronic Aids for the Blind, 28 Crofton Avenue, Orpington, Kent BR6 8DU (day 01-726 4965, Farnborough (0689) 55651 evening)

Essex Voluntary Association for the Blind, 17 High Street, Chelmsford, Essex CM1 1BU (Chelmsford (0245) 352560)

Exhall Grange School, Wheelwright Lane, Coventry CV7 9HP (Coventry (0203) 364200)

Express Reading Service, 79 High Street, Tarporley, Cheshire CW6 0AB (Tarporley (08293) 2115 or 2729)

Family Fund, PO Box 50, York YO1 1UY (York (0904) 21115)

Foundation for Audio Research & Services for Blind People, 12 Netley Dell, Letchworth, Hertfordshire S96 2TF (Letchworth (04626) 74052)
Equipment and Service, Audio Resource Centre, 'St James', Pimlico, near Hemel Hempstead, Hertfordshire HP3 8SJ (Kings Langley (09277) 63564)

Gardner's Trust for the Blind, 46/47 Chancery Lane, London WC2A 1JB (01-242 2287)

Gift of Thomas Pocklington, 20 Lansdowne Road, Holland Park, London W11 3LL (01-727 6426)

Guide Dogs for the Blind Association, Alexandra House, 9/11 Park Street, Windsor, Berkshire SL4 1JR (Windsor (075 35) 55711)

Hypoguard Ltd, Dock Lane, Melton, Woodbridge, Suffolk TP12 1PE (Woodbridge (03943) 7333/4) (supplier for blind diabetics)

International Glaucoma Association, Kings College Hospital, Denmark Hill, London SE5 9RS (01-274 6222 Ext. 2453)

Jewish Blind Society, 1 Craven Hill, Lancaster Gate, London W2 3EW (01-262 3111)
Day Centre, Robert Zimbler House, 91-3 Stamford Hill, London N16 5JP (01-800 5672)

Library Association, 7 Ridgmount Street, London WC1E 7AE (01-636 7543)

Library of Congress, National Library Service for the Blind & Physically Handicapped, 1291 Taylor St. N.W. Washington DC 20542, USA (Tel. (202) 287 5100)

London Association for the Blind, 14-16 Verney Road, London SE16 3DZ (01-732 8771)

Mary Sheridan Unit, Borocourt Hospital, Wyfold near Reading, Berkshire RG4 9JD (Checkendon (0491) 680541)

Moon Branch, Royal National Institute for the Blind, Holmesdale Road, Reigate, Surrey RH2 0BA (Reigate (073 72) 46333)

Multiple Sclerosis Society, 286 Munster Road, London SW6 6AP (01-381 4022)

Muriel Braddick Foundation, 14 Teign Street, Teignmouth, Devon TQ14 8EG (Teignmouth (06267) 6214)

National Association for Deaf/Blind and Rubella Handicapped Children, 12a Rosebery Avenue, London EC1R 4TD (01-278 1771) Manor House Hostel, 72 Church Street, Market Deeping Nr. Peterborough PE6 8AL (Market Deeping (0778) 344921)

National Association of Industries for the Blind and Disabled, Triton House, 43a High Street South, Dunstable, Bedfordshire LU6 3RZ (Dunstable (0582) 606796)

National Association of Orientation and Mobility Instructors (NAOMI), Hon. Sec. Mrs J. Raine, Wallstone Cottage, Alton, Chesterfield, Derbyshire S42 6AR (Chesterfield (0246) 590542)

National Association of Technical Officers for the Blind, Hon. Sec. Mrs P. Shenton, 34 Panmure Road, London SE26 (01-699 2395)

National Bureau for Handicapped Students, 40 Brunswick Square, London WC1N 1AZ (01-278 3459)

National Children's Bureau, 8 Wakley Street, London EC1V 7QE (01-278 9441)

National Deaf/Blind Helpers League, 18 Rainbow Court, Paston Ridings, Peterborough PE4 6UP (Peterborough (0733) 73511)

National Federation of the Blind, Secretary, Mrs Muriel Brain, 45 South Street, Normanton, West Yorks, WF6 1EE (Wakefield (0924) 892146)

National League of the Blind and Disabled, 2 Tenterden Road, Tottenham, London N17 8BE (01-808 6030)

National Library for the Blind, Cromwell Road, Bredbury, Stockport SK6 2SG (061-494 0217)

National Mobility Centre, 22 Melville Road, Edgbaston, Birmingham B16 9JT (021-454 6870)

North London Homes for the Blind, Honeywood House, Station Road, East Preston, Sussex (Rustington (09062) 70339)

North Regional Association for the Blind, Headingley Castle, Headingley Lane, Leeds LS6 2DQ (Leeds (0532) 752666)

Optical Information Council, Walter House, 418-422 Strand, London WC2R 0PB (01-836 2323)

Parents Telephone Service: advice for blind parents and the parents of blind children (Northampton (0604) 407726)

Partially Sighted Society, Secretariat Office: Breaston, Derby DE7 3UE (Draycott (03317) 3036) General enquiries, information and personal advice.
Business office: 40 Wordsworth Street, Hove, East Sussex BN3 5BH (Brighton (0273) 736053). Printing and enlargement services, publications and aids.

Peppard Trust, c/o Dr K.P. Murphy, Audiology Unit, Royal Berkshire Hospital, London Road, Reading, Berkshire RG1 5AN (Reading (0734) 85111)

Queen Alexandra College – see Birmingham Institution for the Blind

Recording for the Blind, Inc., 215 East 58th Street, New York, NY 10022 (New York, USA (212) 751-0860)

Research Centre for the Education of the Visually Handicapped, Selly Wick House, 59 Selly Wick Road, Birmingham B29 7JE (021-471 1303)

Research Unit for the Blind, University of Warwick, Coventry, West Midlands CV4 7AL (Coventry (0203) 24011 Ext. 2162)

Richmond Charitable Trust – see Royal National Institute for the Deaf

Royal Association for Disability and Rehabilitation (RADAR), 25 Mortimer Street, London W1 (01-637 5400)

Royal National College for the Blind, College Road, Hereford HR1 1EB (Hereford (0432) 65725)

Royal National Institute for the Blind, 224/6/8 Great Portland Street, London W1N 6AA (01-388 1266)

Royal National Institute for the Blind, Braille House, 338 Goswell Road, London EC1 (01-837 9921) (for Students Braille and Tape Libraries, Reference Library and Short Document Service)

Royal National Institute for the Blind Commercial College, 5-6 Pembridge Place, London W2 4XD (01-229 6673)

Royal National Institute for the Deaf, 105 Gower Street, London WC1E 6AH (01-387 8033)
Poole Mead (hostel for deaf/blind), Watery Lane, Twerton on Avon, Bath BA2 1RN (Bath (0225) 332818)

Royal School for the Blind, Highlands Road, Leatherhead, Surrey KT22 8NR (Leatherhead (03723) 73086)

Royal School for Deaf Children, Victoria Road, Margate, Kent CT9 1NB (Thanet (0843) 27561 (special unit for deaf/blind children)

St Dunstan's Organisation for Men and Women Blinded on War Service, 191 Old Marylebone Road, London NW1 5QN (01-723 5021)

Society for Blind Lawyers, Secretary: Jeremy Browne, 33 Cornfields, Boxmoor, Hemel Hempstead, Hertfordshire HP1 1UA (Hemel Hempstead (0442) 64355 (day) 47627 (evening)

Scottish Braille Press, Craigmillar Park, Edinburgh EH16 5NB (031-667 6230)

Scottish National Federation for the Welfare of the Blind, 8 St Leonards Bank, Perth PH2 8EB (Perth (0738) 26969)

Scottish National Institution for the War-Blinded, 50 Gillespie Crescent, Edinburgh, Lothian EH10 4HZ (031-229 1456)

Southern and Western Regional Association for the Blind, 55 Eton Avenue, London NW3 3ET (01-586 5655)

Star Housing Association, Chairman: D.R. Kettle, 326 Craven Park Road, London N15 6AN (01-802 1866)

Talking Newspaper Association of the United Kingdom, c/o Mrs J. Deaper, 4 Southgate Street, Winchester, Hampshire SO23 9EF (Winchester (0962) 65570)

Tape Recording Service for the Blind, 48 Fairfax Road, Farnborough, Hampshire GU14 8JF (Farnborough (0252) 47943)

Telephones for the Blind Fund, Mynthurst, Leigh near Reigate, Surrey (Norwood Hill (0293) 862546)

Telesensory Systems Inc., 10 Barleymow Passage, Chiswick, London W4 4PH (01-994 6477)

Torch Trust for the Blind, Torch House, Hallaton, Market Harborough, Leicestershire LE16 8UJ (Hallaton (085 889) 301)

Toy Library Association, Seabrook House, Wyllyotts Manor, Darkes Lane, Potters Bar, Hertfordshire EN6 2HL (Potters Bar (0707) 44571)

Ulverscroft Large-Print Books, The Green, Bradgate Road, Anstey, Leicester LE7 7FU (Anstey (053 721) 4325)

Visual Impairment Association, Membership Secretary: Fred Hodson, 52 Linskill Terrace, North Shields, Tyne and Wear NE30 2EW (Work Newcastle (0632) 574388, home (0632) 583635)

Voluntary Sonic Travel Aid Instruction Centre for the Blind, 22 West Way, South Lancing, West Sussex BN15 8LX (Lancing (090 63) 64474)

Voluntary Transcribers Group, Hon. Sec. A.C. Hackshaw, 4 Shreenwater Cottages, Old Hollow, Mere, Wiltshire BA12 6EB (Mere (0747) 860573)

Wales Council for the Blind, Oak House, 12 The Bulwark, Brecon, Powys LD3 7AD (Brecon (0874) 4576)

Women's Royal Voluntary Service, 17 Old Park Lane, London W1Y 4AJ (01-499 6040)

Wormald International Sensory Aids, 7 Musters Road, West Bridgford, Nottingham NG2 7DP (0602 865 995)

Audio-visual aids

The audio-visual aids listed below are those which are particularly relevant to the topics discussed in this book. Comprehensive lists of films dealing with the deaf-blind can be obtained from the National Association for Deaf-Blind and Rubella Handicapped, whilst the Royal National Institute for the Blind can supply lists of films covering other aspects of blind welfare.

Visual Handicap: Staff Development Package 5 video-tapes together with resource material and simulation exercises. Designed for local authority staff in-service training schemes but suitable also for volunteer training schemes.
   Contact: The Welsh Office, Cathays Park, Cardiff CF1 3NQ (tel. Cardiff (0222) 825111)

Problems of the Blind 8 cassette tape/slide programmes compiled by Jill Allen, a blind housewife, which describe her reactions to sudden visual loss and the ways in which she has dealt with housework, cookery and mobility problems as well as those of motherhood.
   Contact: Southern and Western Regional Association for the Blind.

The Visually Handicapped 4 cassette tape/slide programmes produced by Camera Talks Ltd., which deal with the meaning of blindness, growing up with a handicap, advancing years, and a change of life.
   Contact: Southern and Western Regional Association for the Blind.

The Vision of the Blind 16mm. Colour. 50 mins. A BBC Horizon film which concentrates on the use and value of residual vision.
   Contact: Southern and Western Regional Association for the Blind.

Visual Defects Simulations 16 slides produced by Warwick Research Unit for the Blind to simulate the effect of seven eye conditions. A booklet describing the slides is included. Price £15.
   Contact: Warwick Research Unit for the Blind, University of Warwick, Coventry CV4 7AL (tel. Coventry (0203) 24011).

The Silent Guide 16mm. 16 mins. The teaching of the long cane technique.

Unseen Hazards 16mm. 15 mins. Describes the hazards which needlessly confront the blind pedestrian.

Contact: Royal National Institute for the Blind. The above films are available free on loan.

Out of Sight 16mm. 22 mins. Colour. The special problems of partially sighted children and the ways they can be helped at school, at home and in the community.

Nursery School for the Blind 16mm. 32 mins. Sponsored by the Hampstead Child Therapy Clinic, the film shows how a nursery school helps parents care for their children at home.

Growing Up Without Sight 16mm. 20 mins. Colour. Also sponsored by the Hampstead Child Therapy Clinic, this demonstrates the good functioning that can be achieved by highly intelligent blind children who have no additional handicaps. A method of slowly displacing mannerisms common to the blind to more acceptable activities is also illustrated.

Contact: Concord Films Council, 201 Felixstowe Road, Ipswich, Suffolk IP10 0JZ (tel. Ipswich (0473) 76012).

Communication Limited 16mm. 30 mins. Colour. Deals with deaf-blind and rubella children from young babies to young adults, at home, in units and in schools.

Out of Isolation 16mm. 25 mins. The training of deaf-blind young people.

Contact: The National Centre for Deaf-Blind Children and their Families, 86 Cleveland Road, Ealing, London W13 (tel. 01-991 0513).

Simulating Spectacles Eight sets of spectacles fitted with lenses which create, for a person with normal vision, the effect of different eye conditions. £68.

Contact: Keeler Optical Products (Mr T.L. Glanville), Clewer Hill Road, Windsor, Berkshire SO4 4AA (tel. Windsor (07535) 57177).

Index

Commercial firms and authors of publications are for the most part excluded, as are italicised addresses in the text and the accommodation listed on pages 199–204. Smaller institutions such as schools are entered under the places in or near which they are located. Phrases such as 'of the Blind' are generally omitted.

Choosing a Simple Magnifier

Use this chart wearing reading glasses to find which is the smallest print you can read correctly. Underneath that line is the approximate magnification required to enable ordinary newsprint to be read. For more details of how to use the chart, see page 114, but wherever possible, get professional guidance on choosing a magnifier.

D = Dioptres
X = Magnification
A = Print Size

Look down from

A17 = 10X = 40D

Them upon marshes

A16 = 8X = 32D

Sighed and ice crackled

A15 = 6X = 24D

Quacked on the winter air. It

A14 = 5X = 20D

Was a marsh on one side of the ridge

A13 = 4X = 16D

They could see a wisp of smoke of thirty

A12 = 3X = 12D

Among the trees and a group of buildings far out

A11 = 2.5X = 10D

He went down into the warm starlit water, which ran like a real salmon stream, and struck out for the other side, with his strong arms looking like the limbs.

A10 = 2X = 8D

Now and then they found a cut stump with the marks of an axe on it, but mostly these had been covered over with brambles. This was the answer, so that now

A 9 = 1.6X = 6.4D

Much depends on clear lucid planning. This regretfully does not always have the desired result. Having thus spoken, the old man returned to his planning. This, the old man desired to return his token on the clear

A 8 = 1.3X = 5.25D

And another image came to me, of an arctic hut and a trapper alone with his furs and oil lamp and log fire ; the remains of supper on the table, a few books, skis in the corner ; everything dry and neat and warm inside, and outside the last blizzard of winter raging and the snow piling up against the door. Quite silently a great weight forming against the timber ; the bolt straining in its socket ; minute by minute in the darkness outside the white heap sealing the door, until quite soon when the wind dropped and the sun came

NEWSPRINT.